DR. COLBERT'S

FASTING ZONE

DR. COLBERT'S
FASTING ZONE

DON COLBERT, MD

SILOAM

Most Charisma House Book Group products are available at special quantity discounts for bulk purchase for sales promotions, premiums, fund-raising, and educational needs. For details, call us at (407) 333-0600 or visit our website at www.charismahouse.com.

DR. COLBERT'S FASTING ZONE by Don Colbert, MD
Published by Siloam
Charisma Media/Charisma House Book Group
600 Rinehart Road, Lake Mary, Florida 32746

Visit the author's website at www.drcolbert.com.

Library of Congress Cataloging-in-Publication Data
Names: Colbert, Don, author.
Title: Dr. Colbert's fasting zone / by Don Colbert, MD.
Description: Lake Mary, Florida : Siloam, [2020] | Includes bibliographical references and index.
Identifiers: LCCN 2019041419 (print) | LCCN 2019041420 (ebook) | ISBN 9781629996790 (hardback) | ISBN 9781629996806 (ebook)
Subjects: LCSH: Fasting. | Fasting--Physiological aspects. | Fasting--Religious aspects. | Fasting--Health aspects. | Detoxification (Health)
Classification: LCC RM226 .C64 2020 (print) | LCC RM226 (ebook) | DDC 613.2/5--dc23
LC record available at https://lccn.loc.gov/2019041419
LC ebook record available at https://lccn.loc.gov/2019041420

This book contains the opinions and ideas of its author. It is solely for informational and educational purposes and should not be regarded as a substitute for professional medical treatment. The nature of your body's health condition is complex and unique. Therefore, you should consult a health professional before you begin any new exercise, nutrition, or supplementation program or if you have questions about your health. Neither the author nor the publisher shall be liable or responsible for any loss or damage allegedly arising from any information or suggestion in this book.

Portions of this book were previously published by Siloam as *The Daniel Detox*, ISBN 978-1-62998-647-0, copyright © 2016.

This publication is translated in Spanish under the title *La zona de ayuno del doctor Colbert*, copyright © 2020 by Don Colbert, MD, published by Casa Creación, a Charisma Media company. All rights reserved.

20 21 22 23 24 — 987654321
Printed in the United States of America

"All disease begins in the gut."

—HIPPOCRATES, THE FATHER OF MODERN MEDICINE

CONTENTS

CONTENTS

INTRODUCTION

FASTING HAS BEEN around since the beginning of time, but only in the last twenty to thirty years have we come to better understand (thanks to technology and medical breakthroughs) just how beneficial fasting can be.

Yet even today, we are learning more about the positive impact fasting can have on the body as a whole and on specific parts, specific organs, and even specific cells.

The results may astound you!

To fast is to abstain from food—partially or completely—for a period of time. Fasting has immediate benefits (mentally, physically, emotionally, and spiritually) to your body, including these:

- You usually have more energy! Laziness and lethargy no longer keep you from exercising.

- Cravings are generally under control! Wanting sweets and carbs that lead to extra pounds is common, but fasting usually brings those cravings under better control.

- You often lose weight! A direct result of going without food means your body begins to burn fat instead of sugar, and you usually lose weight.

- Emotions are usually in check! Anger and rage that may send you into a frenzy in traffic or cause you to say hurtful things to your loved ones can be directly reduced by fasting.[1]

- Your health improves! From head to toe, your body's overall health gets a boost as a result of the detoxing and fasting process.

- You are in control! Loneliness, anxiety, depression, and grief have less power to trigger you to seek comfort in sugary, starchy foods.

- Your brain loves it! Fasting offers greater mental focus, attention, and memory.

- Your gut is happy! Many sicknesses and symptoms stem from an unhappy gut, and fasting improves your gut health significantly.[2] And if your gut is happy, it literally will make you happy!

- Your liver is usually able to detox effectively!

But many more benefits come from fasting and making fasting a part of your lifestyle. I have had thousands of patients over the years apply fasting to their regimen, and the list of health benefits they experienced as a result would fill volumes of books.

Some diseases are stopped cold by fasting. I have seen it many times.

For example, patients with type 2 diabetes and prediabetes get tremendous results from fasting. They also change their diet, exercise, and take a few supplements, but fasting plays a big part in helping their bodies heal. That is just one example. I have countless stories I could tell.

Depending on your health goals or health needs, fasting may be especially effective. It really depends where you are, what you need, and where you are going.

I include a twenty-one-day detox fasting program later in the book. This is ideal for supporting your liver, cleansing and detoxifying your body, and giving a rest to your gut that will benefit you for years to come.

To make the process easier, each day in the twenty-one-day detox comes with dietary guidelines and encouragement for the physical aspects of your fast. That is always time well spent.

Others are looking to fasting as an avenue to lose weight. It can certainly help! I have had many patients use fasting to push their bodies out of the plateau they are in. They have already taken steps to lose weight and have had some success, but sometimes our bodies level off and seem stuck at a certain weight. Either full-day fasting or intermittent fasting is powerful and can give your body the push it needs to kick your fat-burning metabolism into higher gear.

Many patients use fasting for their specific medical needs. They have symptoms of sickness or disease and don't want to throw a prescription at it, though that is what our society as a whole does to "fix" most health problems. Sadly, masking a problem will usually make things worse.

The only way to really fix any health challenge is to fix the root cause. Anything less will usually result in further damage and eventually long-term health problems, and nobody wants that!

Every patient is different, but fasting has a way of helping so many people and their many symptoms that I have come to see it as a viable option for almost all of my patients. Obviously, fasting does not cure every single ailment, but it usually does much to help patients get their health back.

Fasting does take some effort, but your body is worth it. It takes time and energy, but your health is worth it. And it doesn't cost much money, which is always good for the pocketbook.

What's more, fasting is easy to do! Not eating or delaying eating is easy. No, it might not be all that fun, but when you are armed with a plan and understand how it really does benefit your body, fasting can easily become a part of your normal routine.

If you haven't looked at fasting as a tool in your arsenal to improve your life, health, and future, I challenge you to do so. Take a second look at it, especially if you have tried fasting in the past and don't even want to consider it. Things have changed. Fasting today is not what it once was.

With that said, let this book guide, teach, and encourage you as you take steps to improve your health. Good will come of it—it always does!

CHAPTER 1

THE MANY BENEFITS OF FASTING

A S A DOCTOR I have been able to look closely at the various popular methods of fasting. Some of them are good, while others can be downright dangerous.

Fasting is often thought of as taking nothing by mouth. Technically speaking, this is true, but it's not the type of fasting I suggest for detoxification. I consider total fasting—not eating or drinking anything—to be very unsafe. Your body must receive at least two to three quarts of water a day to sustain your life, for you can live for only a few days without water.[1]

Although there are many ways to fast, the kind of fast that will bring about the optimum health benefits described in this book is a partial fast. This type of fasting provides fantastic health benefits. For example:

- Fasting gives a restorative rest to your digestive tract.

- Fasting helps the body's designed healing processes to automatically work by giving them a chance to rest from other activities.

- This rest from "digestion as usual" in turn allows your overburdened liver to catch up with its task of detoxification.[2]

- Your blood and lymphatic system also receive needed cleansing of toxic buildup through fasting.

- Fasting allows your other digestive organs, including the stomach, pancreas, intestines, and gallbladder, a much-deserved rest, which allows your cells time to heal, repair, and be strengthened.[3]

A powerful, natural way to bring relief to your body from the burden of excess toxicity, fasting is also a safe way to heal and prevent degenerative diseases.[4] As you can see from the list above, the primary way that fasting allows your body to heal is by giving it a rest.

THE PRINCIPLE OF REST

As with all living things, you need to rest. Sleeping is not the only kind of rest you need. Your digestive system and other organs need a rest from their work as well.

This understanding of the human need for rest is not new to mankind. God introduced the principle of a Sabbath rest to His ancient Jewish nation. It is one of the Ten Commandments (Exod. 20:8). Israel was given specific instructions regarding this divine command to work six days and to rest on the seventh day of each week.

This principle of rest was important as well to their agricultural system. The Israelites were commanded to allow their fields to lie fallow every seventh year to give the soil the rest it needed to reestablish its own mineral and nutrient content. (See Leviticus 25:1–7.)

Today a decreasing number of modern farmers are following this biblical agricultural principle of resting the soil.[5] As a result, the soil has become depleted of some of the minerals and other nutrients that our bodies crave for health. And chemical fertilizers do not succeed in giving us the abundant mineral content of healthy soil.[6]

It is interesting to note that in the animal kingdom, it is a natural habit to seek rest and to abstain from food, especially when the animal is sick or injured. A sick animal refuses to eat and finds a place to rest where it can lap up water and be safe. Some animals hibernate, resting for an entire season without eating.

Rest is also a powerful principle of healing for the human body and psyche. Every night as you sleep, you are providing refreshing rest for your mind and body, which aids health in a tremendous way. Sleep deprivation is a commonly known form of torture, emphasizing the fact of our innate need for rest.

Fasting may be considered an internal rest for the body, allowing it to restore stamina and energy to vital organs by activating the marvelous self-cleansing system with which it is designed.

Your Body's Natural Detox System

To help convince you of the potentially healing benefits of fasting, let me explain briefly the marvelous natural detoxification system God designed for your body. Proper understanding of the innate healing power resident in your body will help you appreciate the phenomenal benefits of fasting.

The hardest-working organ in the body is the liver. Weighing about three pounds, it is also the largest organ inside the body, about the size of a football. It is designed to perform about five hundred functions for the health of the body. Let's look at several of them:

- filtering your blood to remove toxins such as viruses, bacteria, and yeast

- storing vitamins, minerals, and carbohydrates

- processing fats, proteins, and carbohydrates

- producing bile to break down fats for digestion

- breaking down and detoxifying the body of hormones, chemicals, toxins, and metabolic waste

In just one minute your liver can filter about 1.5 quarts of the four to six quarts of blood your body contains. To appreciate the magnitude of this feat, you could compare your liver to the filter in a swimming pool. The filter would need to clean half the pool's water every minute to keep up with what your liver can do. What an incredibly powerful filter your liver is! If it is working efficiently, it can filter out most of the bacteria and other toxins in your blood before sending the cleansed blood back into circulation.

Every day your liver produces about a half quart of bile, which helps to digest dietary fats, breaking them down into a form that can be used as fuel for the body. The bile also functions to eliminate toxins from your body, flushing them out through your colon. For a more complete discussion of these important detoxifying functions of your liver, please read my book *Toxic Relief*.[7]

Unfortunately when this natural filter gets overwhelmed with toxins, it cannot function well, much as a dirty air filter in your car cannot remove dirt from the air. Your liver may get overloaded with toxins from food and water; from food allergies; from bacteria and other microorganisms; from toxins in the air, home, or workplace; and from free radicals produced internally in the liver by the detoxification process itself.[8] Like dust and dirt that accumulate in your air filter, these toxins make the liver work too hard; eventually it may not function efficiently. That is why fasting becomes important, to allow the liver to rest and catch up with its cleansing duties.

Some signs of liver toxicity include the following:

- pallid, yellowish skin
- a coated tongue
- bad breath
- skin rashes
- poor skin tone
- altered or bitter taste in your mouth
- dark circles under the eyes
- yellow discoloration of the eyes
- body odor
- itchy skin

A healthy liver is vital to your overall health. You should do everything you can to keep this champion prizefighter healthy and working at peak efficiency. Fasting is a wonderful way to improve the efficiency of your detoxification system. The first twenty-one days of my fasting program, presented in chapter 7, are designed to provide you with a nutritional program to support and strengthen your liver.

Restoring a healthy GI tract

Have you ever worked on a computer that was overloaded with files, programs, and unnecessary junk? If so, you realize that as a result of being overloaded, your computer works slower and slower, perhaps finally giving up the ghost and refusing to work altogether. Your GI tract can suffer a partial shutdown in a similar way as a result of overloading it with too much junk food.

When people consistently overeat or consume an inadequate amount of fiber, they are placing an enormous strain on their GI tract. Even worse, many people do their overeating late at night, which does not allow the GI tract to rest even when they go to bed; it is still digesting all that "food." Ideally one should fast at least twelve hours every night or not eat anything after dinner until breakfast the next morning.

The small intestine has been designed for several major functions to maintain your health:

- It acts as an organ of digestion and absorption of nutrients to fuel your body's energy level.

- It becomes a protective barrier to keep your body from absorbing toxic materials and other undesirable matter, such as large molecules of undigested food.[9]

- It allows ready absorption of needed nutrients, such as triglycerides from the digestion of fats, sugars from the digestion of carbohydrates, amino acids and di- and tripeptides from the digestion of proteins—all vital compounds needed to ensure your health.

The Physical Benefits of Fasting

In the next chapter we will discuss the specific physical conditions that usually can be reversed or prevented through regular fasting, but here are some of the general benefits your body will enjoy.

Increasing energy and mental clarity

A wonderful benefit of cleansing the body through proper fasting is increased energy levels. Cellular toxins and free radicals impair the mitochondria (the energy factories in each cell), hindering them from producing energy effectively.[10] As a result, you may suffer fatigue, irritability, and lethargy. But when you fast, you allow your cells to shed many toxins and allow your mitochondria to repair so they can again produce the energy you need.[11] Along with increased energy, you will most likely enjoy improved mental functioning as your body cleanses, repairs, and rejuvenates its cells, including those in your brain.[12]

Boosting your immune system

Short-term fasting will also boost your immune system, which will help prevent disease and illness and give you a longer, healthier life. Along with an improved quality of life, you will discover that fasting even makes you look better. Your skin usually will eventually become clearer, giving you radiance you have not known since your youth.[13] The whites of your eyes will usually become clearer—they may even sparkle.

Restoring nature's delicate balance

When your body's tissues are too acidic, precious minerals are lost in the urine and cells may become less permeable, which means they are unable to excrete waste products effectively. In a sense your cells become constipated; they may be full of metabolic waste and cannot eliminate it efficiently. As the cells become more and more toxic, free-radical activity increases, and the toxic overload continues to build until your body starts to deteriorate and degenerative diseases occur.[14]

However, fasting brings back the natural balance. It alkalinizes and raises the pH of the tissues. This enables the cells to excrete toxins again and begins the process of detoxifying your body from head to toe.

Helping you lose weight

Fasting frees your body not only of disease-causing chemicals but also of toxic fat.[15] If you are overweight and even significantly obese, one of the truly wonderful and healthful benefits of partial fasting is that it can help bring your body back to the normal, healthy size that God intended. A regular, sensible fasting or detox program can slim you down very quickly, and you will also experience the more important benefit of reducing the fatty areas in your body where dangerous toxins and chemicals are usually stored.

CAUTION: WHEN YOU SHOULD NOT FAST

Some health conditions and other situations prohibit fasting for certain individuals. While the following list is not exhaustive, it does include some major conditions that prevent you from fasting. Please consult your physician before considering a fast, regardless of your state of health.

- Do not fast if you are pregnant or nursing.

- Do not fast if you are extremely debilitated or mal-nourished, such as patients with AIDS, severe anemia, or any severe wasting conditions.

- Do not fast before or after surgery, since it may inter-fere with your ability to heal.

- Do not fast if you suffer from cardiac arrhythmia or congestive heart failure.

- Do not fast if you are struggling with mental illness, including schizophrenia, bipolar disorder, severe anx-iety, anorexia nervosa, or bulimia.

- Do not fast if you suffer from severe liver or kidney disease.

- Do not fast if you are a type 1 diabetic.

- Do not fast if you are taking anti-inflammatory medications, aspirin, antidepressants, narcotics, or diuretics. (Medications such as thyroid hormones and hormone replacement therapy are safe to take during a fast. Always consult your physician before fasting if you are taking any medication.)

- Do not fast if you are taking prednisone. You will need to first wean off this medication slowly under a doctor's supervision. (You may continue to take low doses of hypertension medications during a fast as long as you are monitored by a physician. However, this does not include diuretics.)

As a physician, I try to help wean my patients off most of their medications prior to supervising a fast for them. If your physician cannot wean you off your medications, then it may be safer to stay on the cleansing and detox fast outlined in chapter 7.

For any extended fast I recommend getting a checkup or physical exam by your doctor first. Have him or her do blood work and a baseline EKG. I normally perform a comprehensive metabolic panel (CMP). This includes kidney function tests (including creatinine and blood urea nitrogen [BUN]), electrolytes, liver function tests, blood sugar, cholesterol, and triglycerides. Along with the CMP, I also perform a complete blood count (CBC), urinalysis (UA), and EKG. These tests should be performed prior to the fast.

During the fast I may perform a CMP and UA once or twice a week, if needed. During each office visit, tell your doctor if you are experiencing any severe weakness, fatigue, or light-headedness. Tell your doctor if you are having any irregular heartbeats. If you develop an irregular heartbeat or pulse, you should be examined by your physician and should probably terminate the fast.

During a fast it is critically important to make sure your blood potassium level remains in the normal range. Low potassium can cause dangerous arrhythmias of the heart and death.[16] That's why it's vital not to take diuretics on a fast.

Juice fasting, however, supplies large amounts of potassium in the fresh-squeezed juices; therefore, it's very unlikely that you will develop low potassium while on a juice fast. Water-only fasts are more likely to cause low potassium levels, especially if you are taking a diuretic medication. Commonly during a fast the uric acid level becomes elevated. This is no cause for concern since it is a normal response of the body to fasting. However, if you have gout, you will need to be monitored more closely by your physician and will need to drink adequate amounts of clean, pure, alkaline water, not tap water.

Children under the age of eighteen should not follow a strict juice fast unless they are closely monitored by a physician.

THE BENEFITS OF HEALTHY EATING

Whether physical conditions prevent you from fasting or not, there are steps everyone can take to improve intestinal health and establish a healthy eating plan. I recommend that, in addition to using the detoxification and fasting program presented in this book, you do the following:

- Always avoid overeating.

- Reinoculate the bowel with supplements containing friendly bacteria: *Lactobacillus acidophilus* for the small intestines and bifidobacteria for the large intestine. These good bacteria can also help prevent damage to the lining of the GI tract, thus maintaining normal intestinal permeability. (See appendix A for recommended supplements.)

- Refrain from excessive eating before bedtime.

- Determine to decrease the stress in your life, especially when eating, by choosing to eat in a relaxed, peaceful atmosphere.

- Stock your pantry with health-first items, and eliminate processed, refined, devitalized, and sugary foods.

- Take a good fiber supplement such as psyllium husk powder or Ketozone fiber. (See appendix A.)

Fasting and establishing healthy eating plans are the first two steps to help you feel and look better than you have in years. However, to keep your body detoxified from the harmful toxins in our world, you will usually have to fast repeatedly to detoxify the body and achieve vibrant health.

Regular fasting is a healthy, biblical way to cleanse your body and soul. In the next chapter we will look at the benefits we can experience when we embark on a health-first lifestyle that incorporates regular fasting.

CHAPTER 2

ADOPTING A FASTED LIFESTYLE

I AM CONFIDENT THAT as you embark on the detox outlined in this book, you will discover that your physical body is an amazing, natural detoxifier. No doubt you will reap many benefits during this detoxification program. But the Fasting Zone is more than a twenty-one-day change; it is a lifestyle change.

In this toxic world it takes more than a passive approach to health care to live long, healthy, active, disease-free lives. It takes wisdom. Throughout this book I present you with the wisdom I have gained as a medical doctor since 1984. As you continue to apply these truths in your future, you will reap the wonderful reward of renewed energy, vitality, and health.

The power of better health through detoxification is yours. I encourage you to pursue your own good health aggressively by looking carefully at your diet and lifestyle. Your own healthy future is in your hands! As you prepare for this short-term, twenty-one-day fast, you also need to prepare for a long-term lifestyle change that puts health first.

As you begin to think about your new health-first lifestyle, remember your body was created to quickly, cleanly, and efficiently deal with any toxin it may encounter. In this chapter I want to introduce you to some of the benefits to your physical body of including periods of regular fasting in your health-first lifestyle. The excessive buildup of toxins contributes to many physical diseases and conditions. Regular fasting is a way to eliminate these toxins and to restore your body to better health.

As you begin, consider the list of some of the conditions and diseases that are often directly linked to a buildup of toxins:[1]

- abdominal bloating
- angina
- asthma
- atherosclerosis
- belching
- cancer
- chronic back pain
- chronic diarrhea
- constipation
- coronary artery disease
- Crohn's disease
- decreased sex drive
- depression
- diabetes
- eczema, chronic acne, and other skin conditions
- fatigue
- fibromyalgia
- food and environmental allergies
- gas
- headaches
- hypertension
- insomnia
- irritable bowel syndrome

- lupus
- memory loss
- menstrual problems
- mental illness
- multiple sclerosis

- obesity
- psoriasis
- rheumatoid arthritis
- ulcerative colitis

Regular fasting holds amazing healing benefits to those of us who suffer illness and disease. From colds and flu to heart disease, regular fasting is a mighty key to healing the body. Let's look at some ways that regular fasting can be used to bring health and healing to a sick body.

FASTING FOR TYPE 2 DIABETES

If you have type 1 diabetes or advanced cancer, you should not fast. However, fasting is extremely effective for most type 2 diabetics.[2] Type 2 diabetics should not fast using fruits or vegetables that have a high glycemic index, such as carrot juice. Instead, you should fast using a high-fiber supplement. (See appendix A.) It is also critically important for diabetics to be on a low-glycemic diet and an aerobic exercise program. For more information on diabetes, see my book *The New Bible Cure for Diabetes*.[3]

Because most individuals with type 2 diabetes also suffer from obesity, fasting is a great way to conquer your weight problems. But remember that fasting for too long can lower your metabolic rate and predispose you to gain even more weight. Short, frequent juice fasts—about three days out of every month—followed up with a healthy eating plan can bring obesity under control quickly and easily. Make sure you use lots of vegetables for juicing rather than using mostly fruit so you don't get too much sugar, and use a high-fiber supplement.

Fasting for Coronary Disease

Fasting is very effective for the treatment of heart disease and peripheral vascular disease. Peripheral vascular disease is simply a buildup of plaque, or atherosclerosis, usually in the arteries of the legs. Periodic fasting may help with plaque removal in the arteries.[4]

While fasting, if you have significant coronary artery disease or peripheral vascular disease, you will find that your cholesterol levels will usually become more elevated on the fast.[5] I tell my patients this happens because the body is in the process of breaking down plaque that is formed in the arteries, so they shouldn't be alarmed.

I always check the blood work before prescribing fasting for my patients. I'm encouraged when I see a dramatic elevation in cholesterol in those with coronary artery disease or peripheral vascular disease while fasting. I know that the fasting is doing its work and usually plaque is being broken down and removed while fasting.

Fasting for Benign Tumors

Undergoing my twenty-one-day fast may help to reduce the size of benign tumors and cysts. These include ovarian cysts, fibrocystic breast changes, lipomas, sebaceous cysts, and even uterine fibroids. If you have advanced cancer, you should not fast. But regular fasting will definitely help you to prevent cancer.

FASTING FOR CROHN'S DISEASE AND ULCERATIVE COLITIS

Fasting is usually very effective for patients with both Crohn's disease and ulcerative colitis.[6] These diseases are usually associated with increased intestinal permeability, toxic overload on the liver, candida overgrowth, dysbiosis (bad bacteria), and numerous food allergies and sensitivities.[7]

Many of my patients with Crohn's disease or ulcerative colitis are very sensitive to all dairy products, nightshades (including jalapeño peppers, potatoes, tomatoes, paprika, and eggplant), and wheat products. In general I find that these individuals are usually extremely sensitive to many forms of sugar. Simple sugars should therefore be totally eliminated from their diet.

Due to their sensitivity to sugar, these people do best on a juice fast with low-glycemic vegetable juices. However, sometimes juicing may aggravate the condition and lead to worsening of diarrhea, and many don't do well with fiber supplements.

If you suffer from Crohn's disease or ulcerative colitis, once your fast is over, eat a plant-based, low-carbohydrate diet. Slowly reintroduce a low-protein, primarily plant-based keto diet with a lot of olive oil and avocado oil into your health-first lifestyle, similar to the twenty-one-day program presented in chapter 7. In addition, keep a good food diary to find out what foods cause food sensitivities, and avoid anything that irritates your GI tract. An alternative is to get an Alcat test (see appendix A).

FASTING FOR AUTOIMMUNE DISEASES

Autoimmune diseases are simply diseases in which the immune system attacks itself. A healthy immune system can tell the difference between normal cells and invader cells. However, in autoimmune diseases the immune system gets confused. It actually produces antibodies that attack and inflame the body's own tissues. Eventually it can damage and even destroy the tissue.

Rheumatoid arthritis and lupus are autoimmune diseases that are often linked to impaired intestinal permeability.[8] Altered intestinal permeability can also happen when you take too many antibiotics that decrease the numbers of friendly bacteria in the intestines or if your intestinal tract has been damaged by anti-inflammatory medications, aspirin, or food allergies or sensitivities.[9]

Autoimmune disease can be aggravated or caused by poor digestion and overconsumption of red meats.[10] Most Americans eat lots of meat and other animal proteins. Our bodies are not equipped to produce the amount of hydrochloric acid and digestive enzymes necessary to digest so much meat. Combine this with the load of stress that most of us live under, which further reduces the amount of the digestive juices such as hydrochloric acid and pancreatic enzymes, and it is no wonder we have an epidemic of bloating, gas, and indigestion!

We eat far too much protein for the amount of hydrochloric acid and digestive enzymes we produce. Therefore, our stomachs and intestines usually can't break down the proteins into the individual amino acids as well as they should. Incompletely digested proteins called peptides, which are much larger than amino acids, are formed. Peptides can be absorbed directly into the bloodstream if you have altered intestinal permeability. Your body may form antibodies to attack these foreign substances. Once again, the body may start to attack itself; if this happens, inflammation will occur.

Too much protein, poor digestion, and altered intestinal

permeability are a recipe for autoimmune diseases such as rheumatoid arthritis and lupus. Rheumatoid arthritis, in particular, is rare in Eastern Mediterranean countries where people eat mainly fruits and vegetables and consume a lot of olive oil.[11] Since the typical American diet tends to increase the inflammation associated with autoimmune diseases,[12] a Mediterranean diet is often recommended for patients with diseases such as rheumatoid arthritis and lupus.[13]

Fasting is one of the most effective therapies for treating or preventing autoimmune diseases,[14] but the earlier in the course of the disease, the better. Juice fasting is especially beneficial in autoimmune diseases. Nevertheless, some physicians have had outstanding results with water-only fasting. If you are going on a fast—especially a water-only fast—for an autoimmune disease, be sure you are carefully monitored by your physician. I do not recommend water-only fasts for individuals who are underweight.

If you have been taking prednisone or other steroid drugs, it is extremely important to wean off these medicines slowly, under medical supervision, prior to fasting. Be sure to watch for signs of adrenal suppression, which include severe weakness and fatigue, rapid heart rate, low blood sugar, and low blood pressure. It may take months to successfully wean off these medications.

After the fast, patients with autoimmune disease should decrease consumption of all animal proteins and avoid dairy products as part of their health-first lifestyle. It is usually helpful to avoid wheat products and nightshades (such as tomatoes, potatoes, peppers, paprika, and eggplant). Instead, choose salads and healthy vegetables with olive oil.

FASTING FOR ALLERGIES AND ASTHMA

Juice fasting is usually extremely helpful if you have allergies or asthma. Your lungs, as well as your entire respiratory tract, are vitally important elimination organs for removing toxins. Fasting often reduces the body's inflammatory reaction to the irritants and toxins that trigger airway hyperactivity.

Allergies—both airborne and food-related—will usually dramatically improve during a fast. Allergic symptoms are improved and sometimes completely disappear.[15] However, it's important to be sure that you are not allergic to any of the juices or foods you will be consuming. Keep a food diary while you are on your fast. Use it to help you avoid anything that may trigger allergic symptoms or symptoms of asthma.

FASTING FOR PSORIASIS AND ECZEMA

I have found that many of my patients with psoriasis and/or eczema suffer from numerous food sensitivities. They usually have increased intestinal permeability and impaired liver detoxification.

It is critically important for those with psoriasis or eczema to fast with juices to which they are not allergic. This is best done by having food sensitivity testing first (such as the Alcat test; see appendix A) or by choosing juices that are not nightshades.

If you have psoriasis or eczema, you may also have yeast overgrowth in your intestinal tract. If you do have yeast overgrowth, parasites, or dysbiosis (bad bacteria), prior to fasting follow a candida diet for at least three months. For more information on candida and yeast overgrowth, refer to my book *The Bible Cure for Candida and Yeast Infections*.[16]

If you find that you do not respond well to a juice fast, you can try a low-lectin fast or fasting friendly food fast (see the appendix), which helps to detoxify the liver. This is an excellent fast for individuals with psoriasis, eczema, fibromyalgia, chronic fatigue, migraine headaches, multiple chemical sensitivities, and autoimmune diseases; it is also good for anyone with impaired detoxification capacity.[17]

Water-only fasting can also be effective for psoriasis or eczema, but it must be closely monitored. If you decide to go on a water-only fast, supplement your fast with detoxifying teas such as dandelion and milk thistle tea.

Before going on any fast for psoriasis or eczema, follow the twenty-one-day liver-support fast that is part one of my twenty-one-day fasting program. If you have psoriasis, you probably have significantly increased intestinal permeability as well as an increased toxic burden on your liver. It is critically important to repair your GI tract and detoxify your liver, with the supplements in appendix A.[18] It is also extremely important to avoid foods to which you are allergic or sensitive.

Patients with eczema are usually sensitive to dairy and peanuts, so these foods need to be eliminated. Patients with psoriasis are many times sensitive to wheat (gluten), nightshades (tomatoes, potatoes, peppers, paprika, and eggplant), red meat, pork, shellfish, dairy, soy, and fried food. Therefore, these foods should be eliminated.

FASTING FOR HYPERTENSION

Do you have high blood pressure? One of the best ways to treat hypertension is to go on a juice fast. Again, make sure you are using plenty of fresh veggies for juicing rather than using mostly fruit. Before your fast, you should first see if you are on a diuretic medication, and if you are, ask your doctor for a safer medication to take during your fast.

Monitor your blood pressure daily while on the fast, and if your blood pressure is normal or low, your doctor may decide to stop the medication or lower it. I have found that when many patients fast and lower their salt intake and stop consuming wheat and corn products, their blood pressure usually drops ten to twenty points, sometimes more. Increase the amount of clean, pure alkaline water (not tap water) you drink to at least 1.5 to 2 quarts a day. Follow the directions for the detoxification fast outlined in this book and the instructions in my book *The New Bible Cure for High Blood Pressure*.[19]

FASTING FOR COLDS AND FLU

When you come down with a cold or flu, fast by drinking plenty of alkaline water and fresh low-glycemic vegetable juices, and get plenty of rest. This will help your system to expel toxic materials through the mucus it creates. Let your fever burn up your infection too. Don't rush to the doctor and take a lot of medications to halt the symptoms. Some of them are important for detoxification.

However, if you have a fever over 102 degrees, you should be examined by a physician. If your fever is greater than 101 degrees and persists for longer than a few days, you should also be examined by a physician. For children, seek medical attention sooner.

You can overcome many infectious diseases like colds and flu by eliminating all dairy products. Also eliminate mucus-forming or mucus-thickening foods such as eggs and processed grains, especially wheat and corn.[20] These grains include pancakes, cereals, doughnuts, tortillas, white bread, crackers, corn chips, pretzels, bagels, white rice, gravies, cakes, and pies. In addition, cut out consumption of margarine, butter, and other saturated, hydrogenated, and processed oils. Also avoid sweets such as candies, cookies, cakes, pies, doughnuts, and so forth.

When you are sick, don't instantly turn to antibiotics. Antibiotics can provide powerful help when you are very ill with a bacterial infection. But the overuse of antibiotics can harm you and has created resistant strains of bacteria. Realize that antibiotics will not treat viruses, which cause the vast majority of infections.

Many doctors prescribe antibiotics for colds and flus that do not even respond to antibiotics. If you have had a fever as described earlier, go see your doctor. But don't insist on getting an antibiotic unless he or she strongly recommends it. For more information, refer to *The Bible Cure for Colds, Flu, and Sinus Infections.*[21]

Let your body's own immune system be your first defense against infections. Overusing antibiotics often creates yeast and bad bacteria overgrowth in the intestinal tract, an increased risk of developing impaired intestinal permeability, and an increased toxic burden on the liver.[22]

We've considered some of the amazing physical results we can experience through regular fasting. Let's go now and take a look at how our everyday lives get built up with all kinds of exterior and interior toxins that can lead to poor health.

CHAPTER 3

A WORLD FILLED WITH TOXINS

W̲E̲ L̲I̲V̲E̲ I̲N̲ a toxic world—one that is taking a heavy toll upon our bodies every day, whether we know it or not. Technological advances since the Industrial Revolution have resulted in dangerous chemicals and pollutants finding their way into our streams, soil, and air—toxins that enter and build up in our bodies, causing toxicity and, eventually, disease. Every day we are exposed to many types of toxins, and some are slowly accumulating in our bodies.

These toxins have changed our environment—around us in our world and within our bodies. For example, at this moment all of the following are true:

- Practically everyone has lead stored in his or her bones.[1]

- Small amounts of DDT or its metabolite DDE are usually found in your fatty tissues.[2]

- Chemicals in tap water are now a major problem in the United States due to pollution.[3]

- Each year industries release about ten million tons of toxic chemicals into the air.[4]

- Pesticides have been linked to brain cancer, prostate cancer, leukemia, and lymphoma.[5] They are sprayed on our produce and are present in higher concentrations in fatty cuts of meat and high-fat dairy products such as butters and cheese.

SICK AND TOXIC

Lead, a soft, malleable metal, is utilized in building materials, vehicle batteries, bullets, pottery glaze, and other products. Because of its long-term and widespread use, lead has affected our entire planet through airborne contamination. It has been found in remote areas around the globe, from the Arctic ice cap to Antarctica.[6]

Lead, mercury, and other metals and chemicals that have polluted much of our water, food, and air are nonbiodegradable, meaning they do not easily break down to less harmful forms. And it isn't just our earth that finds it hard to break down these chemicals. It is also difficult for our bodies to detoxify or eliminate them efficiently. Many times we lack the enzymes required to metabolize them. Thus, these chemicals become stored in our bodies. "It has been established that we have five hundred to seven hundred times more lead in our bones than our ancestors did."[7]

If our earth is sick and toxic, then there is a very good chance that most of us will eventually be sick and toxic. Unfortunately we are usually unable to smell, taste, see, or sense most of the toxic chemicals to which we are exposed on a daily basis. As a result, it becomes increasingly difficult to avoid exposure. If we do not cleanse our bodies of these poisons, we will eventually develop fatigue, chronic degenerative diseases, and maybe even cancer.[8] Could all of these toxins in our environment be the reasons why one in eight women in the United States develops breast cancer and one in nine men in the United States develops prostate cancer?[9]

TOXINS IN OUR AIR

Some of the air we breathe is polluted by exhaust from our cars, buses, trains, and planes and by emissions from industrial sites, waste disposal, and more. Carbon monoxide is one of six primary air pollutants monitored by the US Environmental Protection Agency (EPA).[10] Most carbon monoxide comes from fuel. This dangerous gas has been directly linked to heart disease.[11]

Heavy metals and other pollutants are emitted from smelting plants, oil refineries, and incinerators. Ground-level ozone is the main chemical offender in smog. It irritates the eyes as well as the respiratory tract. The smog and air pollution in some of our major cities can be so high at times in the summer months that residents are warned against exercising outside. The air can become so thick with chemicals that at times it can be difficult to see.

We can live for weeks without food and days without water, but only minutes without air. If the air we are inhaling contains smog, chemicals, carbon monoxide, heavy metals, and other pollutants, then it passes into our noses, into our lungs, and on through our bloodstream. With each breath, toxic chemicals are actually being pumped by the heart to every cell in our bodies via the bloodstream.

Toxins in Our Food and Land

Pesticides continue to be sprayed onto our land, subsequently making their way into our food supply, only to become stored in fatty tissues such as the brain, breasts, and the prostate gland. Every year over 1.1 billion pounds of pesticides and herbicides are sprayed on the crops in America that make up our food supply.[12] The farmers who work closely with these chemicals are at a greatly increased risk of developing certain cancers, especially brain cancer, prostate cancer, leukemia, and lymphoma.[13] Some of these dangerous substances are known to "last in the soil for a very long time, potentially for hundreds of years."[14]

DDT is an extremely dangerous poison that was banned in 1972 due to its devastating effect on wildlife, causing multiple abnormalities in the eggshells of many birds and deformities of reproductive organs of many other animals. Bald eagles, condors, and alligators were among the animals that developed deformities, and their populations decreased dramatically.

Nevertheless, detectable residues of DDE—a derivative of DDT—are still present in most American people.[15]

Pesticides have been linked to a lower sperm count in men and to higher amounts of xenoestrogen in women.[16] Xenoestrogen is a chemical counterfeit of estrogen that fools the body into accepting it as genuine estrogen. This estrogen disrupts the signaling and function of the estrogen made by the ovaries.[17] When estrogen increases, a woman's hormones can become severely imbalanced, leading to symptoms of PMS, fibrocystic breast changes, and potentially endometriosis. It can even have a stimulating effect on breast cancer and endometrial cancer.[18]

No doubt you have tried to wash off a shiny red apple or a dark green cucumber only to find it was covered with a layer of waxy film that was nearly impossible to wash off. Growers do this on purpose. The wax keeps the produce from dehydrating by sealing in water and makes the fruit or vegetable look bright, shiny, and healthy.

Most of these waxes, however, contain powerful fungicides that have been added to keep the food from spoiling, and they may trap pesticides inside the produce.[19] If you want to stay healthy, remove these waxes or buy organic produce that does not contain the waxes.

Because pesticides are usually found in animal feed, our meat supply ends up tainted with pesticides too. Pesticide chemicals accumulate in the fatty tissues of the animals we eat.[20] When we bite into a fatty piece of steak, a greasy hamburger, sausages, bacon, butter, and cream, we are ingesting even more pesticide residues. Our bodies are designed to eliminate the toxins we eat. But when pesticides are not broken down and eliminated from the body, they usually become stored in its fatty tissues.

The body easily absorbs pesticides through the skin by direct contact, the lungs by breathing them in, and the mouth by ingestion. Even though the body is designed to eliminate such dangerous poisons, the sheer amount of them that we encounter daily is far more than our bodies were ever designed to deal with.

Therefore, pesticides, their metabolites, and other dangerous toxins eventually build up in our bodies over time. And the greater the buildup, the more difficult it becomes for the body to eliminate them. When such a residue of pesticides builds up in the body, we can experience the following symptoms or diseases:[21]

- allergies
- Alzheimer's disease
- anxiety
- arthritis
- autoimmune diseases
- cancers such as brain, breast, and prostate cancer[22]
- dementia
- depression
- fatigue
- fibromyalgia
- insomnia
- memory loss
- multiple chemical sensitivity
- Parkinson's and other neurodegenerative diseases
- psychosis and other forms of mental illness[23]

TOXINS IN OUR WATER

Most chemicals that have been emitted into our air, sprayed on our farmlands, or dumped in our landfills will eventually end up in our water. Rains wash these chemicals out of the air and off our land into our lakes and rivers.

Nitrates from pesticides, herbicides, and fertilizers eventually end up in underground aquifers. The toxins gathered in chemical waste sites and dump sites, including landfills, can also eventually seep into our water supplies and contaminate them. Even underground storage tanks that hold gasoline can leak into the groundwater. Rainstorms can actually wash these toxic chemicals into streams and larger bodies of water. Sooner or later they may find their way into our drinking water supply.

Groundwater supplies drinking water for approximately 38

percent of the people in America.[24] Often municipalities treat groundwater with aluminum to remove organic material, and traces of aluminum remain in the drinking water.

Most cities also add fluoride to their drinking water. Fluoride partially inhibits many enzymes in the body, interferes with vitamin and mineral functions, and is linked to calcium deposits and arthritis.

Chlorine is also added to the water to kill microorganisms. Chlorine can combine with organic materials in the water to form trihalomethanes, which are cancer-promoting substances. We actually increase our risk of developing bladder and rectal cancer by drinking chlorinated tap water. In fact, the risk increases as our intake of chlorinated water increases.[25]

Although chlorine kills most bacteria, including the beneficial bacteria in our GI tracts, it does not kill parasites and has a moderate effect on viruses.[26] Parasites include helminths (worms), arthropods (ticks, mites, and other bugs), and protozoa such as amoeba, giardia, and cryptosporidium. Giardia is one of the major causes of diarrhea in day care centers and contaminates many of the lakes and streams in America. It may be showing up in water supplies more often than we think.

An outbreak of the microorganism cryptosporidium in Milwaukee's water supply in 1993 killed sixty-nine people and sickened over four hundred thousand.[27] Some observers believe that certain outbreaks of intestinal flu may actually be caused by such microorganisms in tap water.

INDOOR AIR POLLUTION

Indoor air pollution is often even more dangerous to your health than what you inhale outside. Most people spend about

90 percent of their time inside homes, office buildings, restaurants, factories, and school buildings. Indoor toxins, chemicals, mold toxins, and bacteria get trapped and circulated throughout the heating and air-conditioning systems of these structures and may create a much greater health risk.

Today's buildings are much more airtight and well insulated than they were years ago, making them vaults for germs, bacteria, and chemical toxins. New buildings are the worst. Building materials emit gases into the air through a process known as off-gassing.[28] Paints release solvents such as toluene and formaldehyde. Both new carpets and pressed-wood furniture release formaldehyde into the air as well. Additionally, off-gassing may occur from fabrics, couches, curtains, carpet padding, glues, and more.

High amounts of volatile organic compounds can also be found in offices. These compounds are emitted from copying machines, laser printers, computers, and other office equipment. They cause headaches; itchy, red, and watery eyes; sore throats; dizziness; nausea; and concentration problems.[29]

Airborne mold, bacteria, and fungi such as yeasts can also cause pollution indoors. Many, if not most, air-conditioning units and heating systems contain some amount of mold. The spores from that mold can travel throughout a building. Mold grows wherever dampness is found, which makes air-conditioning units incubators for it. Damp homes breed not only mold but also dust mites. Dust mites are the most common airborne allergy.

Another powerful offender is cigarette smoke. The smoke from a burning cigarette as it sits lit in an ashtray contains a higher toxic concentration of gases than what the smoker actually inhales.[30] Secondhand cigarette smoke contains about four thousand chemicals, including cadmium, lead, arsenic, tars, radioactive material, dioxin (which is a toxic pesticide), carbon monoxide, hydrogen cyanide, nitrogen oxides, and nicotine.[31]

THE DANGERS OF SOLVENTS

Solvents, which are chemicals used in cleaning products, are everywhere. Solvents dissolve other materials that otherwise would not be soluble in water.

Solvents can stress and eventually injure the kidneys and liver. They can also depress the elaborate central nervous system of our bodies.[32] Like pesticides, solvents are fat-soluble, which simply means they are likely to be stored in our fatty tissues, including the brain, breasts, and prostate gland. Solvents have the ability to dissolve into the membranes of our cells, especially our fat cells, and accumulate there.[33]

Take a look at some common solvents and the problems they cause:

- Formaldehyde is commonly used to make drapes, carpet, particleboard, and even cosmetics. Formaldehyde exposure is associated with nasal cancer, nasopharyngeal cancer, and possibly even leukemia.[34] Exposure to formaldehyde can also cause asthma, headaches, memory lapse, nosebleeds, eye irritation, and other conditions.[35]

- Phenol is widely found in cleaning products such as Lysol and is used to make aspirin and sulfa drugs. Phenol is easily absorbed by the skin and can cause burns, numbness, wheezing, headaches, nausea, and vomiting.[36]

- Benzene is a solvent used in making dyes and insecticides. "Long-term exposure to high levels of benzene in the air can cause leukemia."[37]

- Toluene is similar to benzene and is used for making a variety of different glues and paint thinners. Elevated levels of toluene in the body are associated with arrhythmias of the heart as well as nerve damage.[38]

- Vinyl chloride is used in the manufacture of PVC pipes and plastic food wrappers, and it has been linked to several types of cancers and sarcomas.[39]

- PCBs, which were banned in 1979, have contaminated many of our lakes and streams and are associated with an increased risk of all types of cancer. Several studies have shown significant increase in deaths from gastrointestinal tract cancers and lymphoma in workers who were exposed to PCBs.[40]

As you can see, even our cells, tissues, and organs are being bombarded with toxic chemicals from every direction. We are being exposed to pesticides, solvents, and other chemicals through our food, water, and environment every day.

But we are not hopeless. We do not need to sit passively by while our immune systems break down and diseases develop under the heavy burden. Detoxification is available. We can cleanse our bodies from years of accumulated toxins and their effects by learning to support the body's own elaborate system of detoxification.

CHAPTER 4

A BODY FILLED WITH TOXINS

E VEN IF YOU lived in a perfect, unspoiled environment with no chemicals or poisons, your body would still produce its own toxins. Your body creates many different toxins in an infinite variety of ways just to function.

In a perfect environment, dealing with your body's internal toxins would be a cinch for your liver and excretory system. But your liver, GI tract, organs, and tissues have been bombarded from without and within by far more poisons than they were ever designed to handle. Take a look at some of these toxic enemies:

- If you have had repeated bouts of antibiotics, or even a single bout of superantibiotics, then you could be at risk for developing an overgrowth of dangerous intestinal bacteria and yeast.

- Free radicals are continuously being produced in our bodies every day and, if unchecked, will set the stage for cancer, heart disease, and a host of other potentially fatal diseases.

- Too many sugars, fats, processed foods, fast foods, and other devitalized foods are literally draining the life out of us as they constipate our bodies, introduce toxins, inflame our tissues, and drain us of our nutrient reserves.

- Fried foods, hydrogenated and partially hydrogenated fats, excessive amounts of polyunsaturated fats, and food sensitivities also cause inflammation in the body. We now know that arthritis, autoimmune disease, asthma, cardiovascular disease, Alzheimer's disease, and most cancers are associated with excessive inflammation.

WHEN THE CURE CAUSES THE CRISIS

Without antibiotics we'd be in trouble. Infections that might have snuffed out a life a century ago are little more than a nuisance today. But we are just beginning to get a full picture of the toll the overuse of antibiotics has taken on a generation of users.

Your intestines are filled with good bacteria, such as *Lactobacillus acidophilus* and *bifidus*, which prevent the overgrowth of pathogenic bacteria (bad bacteria) in your intestinal tract. When you take antibiotics, many of your body's beneficial bacteria can be killed. Your good bacteria function like a fire wall to keep pathogenic bacteria and yeast in check. So when antibiotics throw off the balance, the bad bacteria and yeast may grow like a wildfire, out of control with nothing to slow them down or stop them.

Bad bacteria may produce endotoxins, which may be as toxic as almost any chemical pesticide or solvent that enters your body from outside. Overgrowth of bacteria in your small intestines can cause excessive fermentation, just like the fermentation that happens when you leave apple cider outside for too long. This fermentation process creates even more toxins, such as *indoles*, *skatoles*, and amines,[1] and leads to small intestinal bacteria overgrowth (SIBO).

Just like a biblical plague of locusts that ravaged ancient farmlands, yeast overgrowth causes damage to the intestinal lining. Candida albicans is a yeast that releases almost eighty different toxins into the body.[2] Some of the most toxic substances produced by Candida albicans are acetaldehyde and ethanol, which is alcohol. For more information on this topic, refer to my book *The Bible Cure for Candida and Yeast Infections*.

The EPA has concluded that acetaldehyde is probably a human carcinogen, based on studies of its effects on animals.[3] Acetaldehyde is extremely toxic to the brain, even more so than ethanol. It causes memory loss and concentration problems.[4]

When you consider the potential danger of having strong, devastating poisons created inside your body, you will recognize that the toxins within can do as much or even more damage than environmental toxins.

THE MOLECULAR WARFARE OF FREE RADICALS

While you are going about your daily business, a war is raging inside your body at the molecular level. Free radicals are similar to microscopic shrapnel, machine-gunning through the body, injuring cells and tissues throughout the day. Let me explain.

Picture an atom. It has a nucleus surrounded by electrons.

The nucleus is positively charged, and the electrons are negatively charged. It looks something like the sun with the planets revolving around it.

When you are exposed to air pollution or radiation, when someone blows smoke in your face, or when you ingest alcohol or some other chemical or pesticide, the free radicals created by the toxins can pull one of the electrons out of orbit. When the atom, which is missing an electron, becomes unstable, it grabs an electron from another nearby molecule to replace it, causing a chain reaction.

Free radicals are produced in the body, and in small numbers inside cells, they are actually useful in activating many enzyme and biological reactions.[5] However, toxins such as air pollution, cigarette smoke, pesticides, solvents, and heavy metals cause the production of excessive amounts of free radicals, causing damage to cells, tissues, and organs.

Each of your body's trillions of cells has a protective wrapping around it made of lipids or "fatty" cell membranes. But free radicals, like wrecking balls, can start ricocheting off the cell membranes—eventually damaging intracellular structures such as the mitochondria and nucleus.

When free radicals begin a chain reaction, they must be stopped quickly. Antioxidants rush to the rescue instantly to quench the free-radical fire of activity. Literally hundreds of different compounds function as antioxidants. Many are found in foods and supplements, and others are naturally produced by the body. Many free radicals occur with normal metabolic processes in all cells in the body. Internal antioxidants such as superoxide dismutase, glutathione peroxidase, and catalase work as antioxidants, controlling free-radical production.[6]

But problems occur when the level of free-radical activity gets out of control or if the body has diminished antioxidant reserves. When our bodies are overburdened with free radicals from air pollution, pesticides, solvents, cigarette smoke, sugars, fried foods, and polyunsaturated fats in our diet, then excessive amounts of free radicals ravage our cells. They can actually cause the breakdown of the fats in the cell membranes, ravage the proteins and enzymes, and then eventually damage DNA, causing mutations. These mutations may eventually result in cancer.[7]

A STRATEGY FOR WINNING THE WAR AGAINST TOXINS

You may feel overwhelmed by the monumental battle your cells, tissues, and organs are faced with each day. As you look in the mirror, you may even see some of the results of this war: premature aging, sickness, chronic fatigue, arthritis, cancer, heart disease, and so much more.

The good news is that you don't have to sit by passively while your God-given entitlement to good health is stolen right out from under your nose. Your body is designed with an incredible system of defense that keeps you healthy even under extreme circumstances—and you never have to give it a second thought. But when the battle becomes overwhelming, when toxins pile up inside you over time, your liver and excretory system may eventually become overburdened. They simply cannot keep up.

However, you can choose to step in and even the score. By undergoing my twenty-one-day program of detoxification outlined in chapters 7 and 8 of this book, you can cleanse your body from a lifetime of toxins and discover the health and vitality that come with internal cleansing. You will simply be amazed at how much better you will feel after freeing your body of its toxic burden.

In my practice I have encouraged many of my chronically ill patients to undergo detoxification. The results have been astonishing. Heart disease, diabetes, hypertension, arthritis, chronic fatigue, and many other serious diseases are being absolutely reversed as my patients cleanse their own bodies from toxins. Your health will improve dramatically once those toxins are removed rather than circulated to other areas of the body. Not only will you look better, but you will also feel better and live longer too.

Your Program for Detoxification

Here's an overview of my fasting program:

- You will undergo a three-week partial fast to strengthen and support your liver and improve your elimination through the GI tract.

- You will follow my four-day guidelines for breaking your fast. (Note: I recommend that you go back on the special diet for your liver and GI tract for another two weeks after you complete the fast.)

As you go through this fasting program, you will discover renewed energy, rejuvenated health, and a fresh, glowing sense of vitality that will absolutely astonish you.

However, my fasting program is only one part of a two-pronged solution for dealing with toxins on a regular basis. The second part is making lifestyle changes and establishing a plan to fast periodically in order to continue to cleanse and maintain your health. For you to understand the importance of doing both parts of this program, I want you to face the terrible truth about the American diet.

CHAPTER 5

YOUR GUT HEALTH

OR THE PAST twenty years, countless patients have come in with a similar list of symptoms: feeling bad, constant fatigue, brain fog, chronic infections, loose stools, abdominal bloating, gas, abdominal pain, rashes, and more. In fact, I used to have those same symptoms myself.

The condition I just described is called dysbiosis. It is rampant in this country, and very few doctors are addressing it.

In my efforts to find the cause, I came to find that there were actually many different causes. And the more research I did, the wider the problem became. It was usually a combination of several factors, including these:

- consuming too many antibiotics, for sickness as well as from the foods we eat (Did you know that 70–80 percent of the antibiotics made are given to animals, which we then eat?[1])

- taking anti-inflammatory medications, including aspirin, ibuprofen, and naproxen, and stomach acid inhibitors, such as Prilosec, Nexium, etc.

- consuming excessive alcohol

- experiencing chronic stress

- having recurrent infections

- eating a bad diet

The one place where all these factors crossed was in the gut.

It turns out that the gut is foundational to our health. Fasting's role in regard to gut health is to provide an incredibly effective way to give your gut time to rest, heal, and recharge. And with a gut restoration program, fasting can help remove bad bacteria and increase good bacteria in your gut.

We will discuss this is greater detail. But first, it is important to understand more about your gut and how it plays such an important part in your health, disease prevention, weight loss, and so much more.

What Happens in Your Gut

The gut, comprised of the small and large intestines, has become increasingly prominent over the last twenty years. That is simply because we more fully understand the role the gut plays in our health and well-being.

How could the great physician Hippocrates, who lived from about 460 to 370 BC in Greece, have really known that all disease begins in the gut? Modern medicine is only recently coming to the same conclusion! I now call gut restoration the foundation of health.

Everyone knows the role of the gut is to digest food, absorb the nutrients from that food, and then excrete as waste what is left over. But did you know that your gut also plays a huge role in your immune system? Or that your gut is in constant communication with your brain?

In fact, researchers have found that

- 70–80 percent of your body's total immune cells are found in your gut!

- 95 percent of your body's serotonin (the "happy chemical" that gives you a good mood) is made in your gut!

- one hundred million neurons that communicate with your brain are in your gut![2]

Your gut does all this and so much more. In fact, research from around the world has found that the gut holds as many as one hundred trillion microbes (bacteria). A single drop of fluid from your large intestine contains more than a billion of these bacteria![3]

This directly implies that much of the weight-loss battle is waged in the gut. In fact, in a very interesting study, obesity researchers transferred fecal pellets from fat rodents to the colons of skinny rodents, and the skinny rodents started eating so much that they too became fat. In another case, when rodents received a transplant of microbes related to leanness, the rodents tended "to gain less weight than untreated mice."[4]

How is that possible? It's the microbes in the gut! The gut bacteria play a big role in weight loss and weight gain. This is a new frontier in obesity research that may result in more breakthroughs, allowing us to improve our gut health and to help us lose weight.

In addition to weight-loss challenges, people who are constantly fighting to stay healthy or to avoid depression may also have gut health issues. The gut plays such a big role in so many health-related factors in our lives that I would not be surprised if the gut becomes the focus of many of our most pressing sicknesses and diseases. In fact, one of the new research topics in mental health is psychobiotics, or probiotics that support mental health.

People go to a doctor because they are sick, naturally, but in my experience it is rare for a chronically sick patient to simultaneously have a healthy gut. At least with my patients, almost every disease, illness, or symptom is reflected in the gut.

The goal, then, is to have your gut be as healthy as possible—to remove bad bacteria and support the trillions of good bacteria that live there and play a vital role in every single aspect of your life.

It is actually these trillions of beneficial bacteria that digest much of your food. They are responsible for converting your food into energy that your body then uses. They even make countless enzymes, vitamins, and hormones that your body cannot make by itself.[5]

IT'S A FACT

Food allergies are rare. Only about 4 percent of the US population have an actual food allergy.[6]

In short, without all the beneficial bacteria in our gut, we would all be in trouble. Truth is, we would probably be dead. From birth to the grave, these bacteria help to keep us alive and our immune system strong.

But what we eat and how we treat our bodies have a direct cause-and-effect relationship on our health, immune system, mood, neurological function, and more. Treat your bacteria well, and these trillions of good bacteria will take good care of you. That's what is happening in your gut every moment of every day.

GLUTEN, FOOD SENSITIVITIES, AND ALLERGIES

Though it dominates the airwaves, packaging, books, and restaurants, gluten (a protein found in various grains) is not the only food item causing pain and discomfort. There are countless other things to be concerned about. However, because gluten is so famous these days and because a billion-dollar gluten-free industry now thrives, it's worth talking about gluten and your gut.

Say "gluten" and some people will think celiac disease (an autoimmune disease) or food allergy, while others will think food sensitivity (food intolerance). Which is it? The answer depends on the person's gut.

The least of these three is a food sensitivity or food intolerance. Food intolerances are usually due to a damaged gut (leaky gut). These will usually go away when your gut heals.

Though not life threatening, the symptoms are still never fun. The most common side effects with my patients, in descending order, include these:

- stomachache
- bloating
- joint pain
- gas
- fatigue
- itching

- headache
- diarrhea
- constipation
- heartburn
- rashes
- depression

> ## IT'S A FACT
> *It is estimated that 6 percent of the US population are gluten sensitive.*[7]

If your gut—specifically the trillions of bacteria in your gut—did not like what you fed it, these symptoms are a pretty clear sign that you should stop eating whatever it is you ate.

Why your gut is having the reaction is another question entirely. A few common reasons your gut may be sensitive to a food are the following:

- lack of/insufficient enzymes in the gut to break down the food properly

- chemicals in the food (i.e., sulfites, artificial colors, etc.)

- toxins, including those that naturally occur in the food[8]

- leaky gut or increased intestinal permeability

- dysbiosis (excessive bad bacteria)

Regardless of the cause, the symptoms are pretty hard to miss. You may misdiagnose them, but you won't miss them. They are annoyingly persistent, like a cough that never goes away or a nose that always seems to drip.

Besides gluten, other common foods that may generate a lot of these symptoms are such things as dairy products, eggs, corn, and soy. An easy way to truly know whether someone is sensitive to a food is through the process of elimination.

Fasting is a perfect time to test yourself. After your fast—ideally a three- to twenty-one-day detox fast—you can introduce one food at a time that you have wondered if your body is sensitive toward. After a few days of eating that food, set it aside and try another. It won't take you long to tell because your gut will be quick to show any displeasure.

As for food allergies, in the best case they upset your gut, which then negatively affects your body. In the worst case they can be deadly. In short, allergies can be really bad news for your gut and for you.

This list of food allergy symptoms is painfully real. I see most of these signs come through my office door routinely. If you have experienced these, you know what I'm talking about:

- acne
- anaphylaxis
- asthma
- bloating/excess weight
- brain fog
- canker sores
- coughing
- dark circles under the eyes
- dizziness
- earaches
- eczema/rashes
- fatigue
- headaches/migraines
- hives (urticaria)
- mood swings (anxiety, aggressiveness, irritability)
- shortness of breath
- sinus problems
- skin discoloration
- tight/hoarse throat
- tongue swelling
- vomiting
- weak pulse[9]

Sadly, most people are trained to treat the symptom and not the cause. They will medicate to "treat" their asthma or acne or eczema, but all they have done is mask it. The gut isn't happy, but they keep on eating the foods that caused or aggravated these problems.

Clearly, the best answer is to figure out what food causes the problem and stop eating it. Again, fasting is a great time to begin that elimination process.

Peanut allergies are well known, but many foods, such as these, can cause allergic reactions:

- cow's milk
- eggs
- fish
- nuts (from trees)
- shellfish
- soy
- wheat

A food allergy causes the immune system to kick in, which is what initiates the reaction. Protecting your body from danger, the immune system sees the food as a direct threat to your body.

Whereas a food sensitivity usually involves a delayed reaction occurring hours or even days after eating a specific food that you might be sensitive to, food allergies are different. Usually with a food allergy, your body will feel the impact immediately, on your skin, in your gut, in your lungs, or in your circulatory system. These reactions are nothing to play with.

Gluten falls in both categories—as a food sensitivity as well as an allergen. But it is just one of many foods that people react to. Knowing the differences between sensitivities and allergens is helpful. Even more so is understanding what happens behind the scenes in the gut when these types of foods are eaten.

WHEN THINGS GO WRONG IN THE GUT

Consuming foods you are allergic to or sensitive to causes more inflammation in the gut. As a direct result, the environment in the gut becomes more favorable for bad bacteria, which pushes out the good bacteria, and conditions continue to worsen.

Think of it as a gradual slide toward bad health, obesity, and premature death. This is happening to millions of people across the nation and around the world, but they aren't aware of it.

The symptoms they experience are signs that something is wrong in the gut, and the gut cannot handle it all. Masking the problem doesn't make it go away. It only gets worse and worse over time.

It's called a leaky gut. If you are not familiar with the term *leaky gut*, you soon will be. More and more, medical professionals and researchers are seeing leaky gut as a foundational cause of numerous sicknesses and diseases, especially autoimmune diseases.[10]

If your mind jumped ahead and you are wondering whether fixing the gut could do the reverse, causing the sicknesses and diseases to stop and even go away, you are correct. It does work that way!

Sadly, when it comes to the gut, most people operate by the "If it isn't broken, don't fix it" philosophy.

Among other challenges, failure to fix a leaky gut usually leads to weight gain.

Failure to fix a leaky gut also usually leads to inflammation in the GI tract and throughout the body. This is such a common symptom that many of my patients think it's "normal." But inflammation is not good! It's a clear signal that something is wrong in the gut.

Believe it or not, "inflammation is the root cause of most chronic diseases, including cardiovascular disease, arthritis, Alzheimer's disease, Parkinson's disease, most cancers, autoimmune disease (such as rheumatoid arthritis, lupus, MS, colitis, Crohn's disease), and more."[11]

Failing to fix a leaky gut leads to a lot of unnecessary pain, sickness, ailments, expense, disease, and aging—even to death. One medical doctor wrote, "Although...I originally thought that leaky gut was an isolated condition affecting a few unfortunate individuals, now I am convinced that leaky gut underlies all our disease issues, just as Hippocrates posited."[12]

Without question, fixing a leaky gut should be high on everyone's priority list!

How Does the Gut Leak?

Your body has four points of defense against the many viruses and bacteria out there:

- mucus in your nose and saliva in your mouth

- stomach acid

- beneficial bacteria in your mouth and gut

- the layer of mucus produced in your intestines[13]

Deep down in the gut is where the immune system provides us with the most concentrated amount of nonstop protection. The innate immune system in the gut is the first line of defense. Its job is to stop bad molecules from entering the bloodstream. If the molecules (bacteria, viruses, food components, yeast, toxins, etc.) somehow get through, the adaptive immune system comes to fight the invading molecules by sending antibodies that attack the specific molecules. In fact, the invader molecules are memorized so that if they return, the body can respond more quickly the next time.[14]

But as amazing as the gut is, the lining is only a single cell thick. That's right: the lining of the gut is just one cell thick, yet it has a surface area of 30–40 square meters—the size of a small studio apartment![15] The challenge is keeping those gut cells (enterocytes) tightly bound together and preventing breaches in the gut wall to keep the bad actors out and allow the good nutrition in.

The cells of the gut wall are held together by tight junctions that prevent anything foreign or harmful from breaching the barrier and entering the bloodstream and tissues. The tight junctions are designed to regulate the flow of micronutrients, vitamins, simple sugars, enzymes, fatty acids, amino acids, etc. through the wall and into the body. That's how the absorption of food works, all at the microscopic level.

However, with a leaky gut, what gets through the breaches in the gut wall causes havoc in our bodies.

IT'S A FACT

One common side effect of leaky gut is weight gain.

See the lining of the gut as a football team with every member positioned on the line. When the opposing team's running back breaks through the weak link in the line, scoring a touchdown is inevitable because no linebackers, cornerbacks, or safeties are there to stop him. In a leaky gut, the same football players on the defensive line are standing three yards apart, not lined up in a row shoulder to shoulder, and the harmful substances are like the opposing running back, heading straight into the bloodstream with little to stop them!

Or view it as a damaged coffee filter. If you poke holes in the filter with a fork, your cup of coffee will be full of coffee grounds, similar to the breaches in the gut wall allowing all sorts of toxins and partially digested food into the bloodstream.

With a single-cell wall defense, our gut is much like this. It is exposed to so many foods, medications, stresses, and more that are causing leaky gut, and once the barrier is breached, many health issues and problems arise.

The breaching of the gut wall allows larger molecules, such as proteins and partially digested foods, to enter directly into the bloodstream. Our body is designed to absorb micronutrients such as amino acids, fatty acids, and simple sugars, not full-size proteins, intact carbohydrates, large fats and bacteria, and more.

We are not talking about a single hole in the gut. Rather, we are talking about millions of minute holes that allow bacteria, partially digested food, and toxins into the body.

There is your inflammation!

When you have a leaky gut, inflammation happens in your intestines, and you will react to many more foods. These are not actually food allergies but food sensitivities that happen because the leaky gut lets the wrong things in.

Interestingly, we can now measure the degree of leaky gut that someone has. Zonulin, discovered in 2000 by Alessio Fasano at the University of Maryland School of Medicine, is a protein that helps manage the permeability of the gut wall. When zonulin levels rise, one has leaky gut, or increased intestinal permeability.

So what causes the number of zonulin proteins to increase?

The top two causes are (1) bad bacteria in the gut and (2) gluten in the foods we eat.[16]

This zonulin plays a part in many autoimmune diseases, including celiac disease. People with autoimmune diseases usually have high zonulin levels and therefore a leaky gut.[17]

When the gut wall is compromised, the entire body is at risk. I have collected a list of things for my patients to avoid because of the negative impact on their gut health:

- alcohol (reduce or remove entirely)
- antibiotics
- anti-inflammatory medications, such as aspirin (even baby aspirin), ibuprofen (Advil, Motrin), naproxen (Aleve), etc.
- chlorinated water
- excessive chronic stress
- excessive meats
- gluten
- GMO foods
- high-lectin foods
- many prescription drugs
- processed foods/ sugars
- sugar (and artificial sweeteners)
- ulcer medications

Everything on this list pretty much damages the gut, contributes to inflammation in the gut, gives the bad bacteria in your gut a boost, and reduces all the good bacteria that are working to make your body healthy.

IT'S A FACT

A leaky gut can make your body react to foods you are not even allergic to.[18]

How to Fix a Leaky Gut

The way to heal a leaky gut certainly falls under the "easier said than done" category because there are so many moving parts to the puzzle. But after many years of working with patients to help heal leaky gut, I have discovered three basic steps that everyone with a leaky gut needs to take:

1. Remove the offending foods, medications, and stress.

2. Reinoculate the gut with good bacteria, and rid the gut of bad bacteria.

3. Restore the integrity of the gut (such as through fasting).

This three-step process applies to each different thing that may be causing damage to your gut. For example, if you have been taking anti-inflammatory drugs such as Advil or Aleve for years, then they are probably only masking the problem—and they are causing leaky gut. Eventually you will want to stop. You will need to work on increasing the good bacteria in your gut by taking probiotics and reducing anything else that may be causing gut damage. This naturally decreases the bad bacteria. And then stay away from the drugs that caused the damage in the first place. (See appendix A for probiotic, prebiotic, and fiber recommendations.)

When you strengthen the gut and remove all the things that trigger a leaky gut, you will be amazed at how well your gut heals. Sometimes it happens very quickly. Remove the thorn—usually a food you crave and eat every day, sometimes at every meal—and the body heals.

Fasting usually gives your GI tract a needed break from all things inflammatory. This time-out helps your gut repair, and if you fast regularly, it helps strengthen your gut repeatedly.

I have seen symptoms simply disappear from patients with leaky gut who applied this three-step process and then fasted regularly. The results have been astounding. And usually the gut will heal itself as you keep this process up.

Giving your body good bacteria is also highly recommended. (See appendix A.) Taking some form of probiotic will usually help. Noted medical doctor Robynne Chutkan also suggests prebiotics, which are "non-digestible foods or ingredients that promote the growth of beneficial microorganisms in the intestines" (i.e., green bananas, "onions, garlic, leeks, asparagus, and artichokes"), and synbiotics, which "are a combination of prebiotics and probiotics that are found primarily in fermented foods such as pickles, sauerkraut, kimchi, and kefir."[19]

While you are fasting, take probiotics; then follow your fast with prebiotics and fiber as part of your regular diet.

Keeping your gut healthy is vital to your body's overall health.

CHAPTER 6

PORTION CONTROL

"**D**IET IS A significant factor in the risk of coronary heart dis ease (CHD), certain types of cancer, and stroke,"[1] which are three of the leading causes of death in the United States. Heart disease and cancer caused 44.9 percent of all deaths in 2016.[2]

"Diet also plays a major role in the development of diabetes (the seventh leading cause of death), hypertension, and overweight. These six health conditions incur considerable medical expenses, lost work, disability, and premature deaths—much of it unnecessary, since a significant proportion of these conditions is believed to be preventable through improved diets."[3]

We abuse our bodies in many ways through our poor eating habits, but here are a few of the major abusers in our diets:

- The average American consumes more than 150 pounds of sugar per year. That's the equivalent of about one to two teaspoons of sugar per hour![4]

- Processed foods are grossly deficient in nutrients and contain food additives, sweeteners, flavorings, coloring agents, preservatives, bleaching agents, emulsifiers, texturizers, humectants, acids, alkalis, buffers, and other chemicals. Such foods provide loads of calories with little nutrition.

- Our soil has been robbed of important minerals and nutrients; therefore, the food it produces is nutritionally poor.

- The fat we eat, including excessive saturated fats, excessive polyunsaturated fats, and hydrogenated fats, overtaxes our bodies with thick, sludge-like, yellowish-brown material that encrusts the inside of our arteries, forms plaque, fattens our bodies, elevates our cholesterol, forms stones in our gallbladders, weakens our immune systems, and shortens our lives.[5]

- Fast foods, fried foods, and eating far too much meat while denying our bodies healthful fruits and vegetables are ways in which we abuse our bodies through our diets.

It's easy to see why we're overfed and undernourished. We gorge ourselves with increasing amounts of food to respond to our bodies' cravings for nutrition. After we've eaten, our bodies, even though under a heavy burden of calories, still realize that they never received the nutrients they needed. So our brains send more signals, triggering hunger, which we interpret as the need or desire for even more food. We end up spiraling down into a vicious cycle of overfeeding with empty foods, craving more nutrition, and overfeeding again with even more empty, processed, devitalized, sugary foods.

The end result is ever-expanding waistlines, thighs, and buttocks. We get fatter and fatter, forcing our bodies to groan under the burden of extra pounds. But in terms of actual nourishment, we give our bodies less and less.

We may be actually starving from a nutritional standpoint while at the same time becoming grossly obese. The end result of this merciless abuse of our bodies is disease and death. Sadly, we really are digging our graves with our forks and knives!

As a result of our overindulgences we have an epidemic of heart disease, atherosclerosis, hypertension, diabetes, autoimmune disease, cancer, allergies, obesity, arthritis, osteoporosis, dementia, and a host of other painful and debilitating degenerative diseases.

Junk Food Overload

Americans have been duped into believing that we can continue to exist on junk food day by day and simply add a multivitamin—or a multitude of vitamins—a day to protect ourselves from whatever we have eaten while maintaining excellent health. Taking vitamins and other nutrients while continuing to eat poorly is similar to adding small amounts of oil to keep a car's oil level in normal range but never changing the oil or oil filter while continuing to drive it.

Over the years as I have treated people with degenerative diseases, I have noticed a pattern. Most of these individuals aren't underfed. In fact, most of them are big overeaters. They eat plenty—but they eat all the wrong things. They are overfed and yet completely undernourished. This is particularly true of most people with obesity, cardiovascular diseases, arthritis, type 2 diabetes, migraine headaches, a host of different allergic conditions, psoriasis, rheumatoid arthritis, lupus, and other autoimmune diseases. In fact, to some degree, it appears to apply to nearly all degenerative diseases.

For many of these people, medications won't help. Nor can taking vitamins and nutrients eliminate the cause of the diseases. That's because it is not lack that causes many of these diseases— it is eating too much of the wrong foods.

One of the main causes of degenerative diseases is overconsumption of sugary, fatty, starchy, and high-protein foods—foods that have been processed, fried, genetically modified, and further devitalized. Individuals with these diseases typically take in enormous amounts of empty, fattening calories, but they are not nourishing their bodies.

Taking supplements such as a comprehensive multivitamin with minerals, antioxidants, and so forth is important. However, it is much more important to eliminate (or significantly reduce) consumption of saturated and polyunsaturated (not monounsaturated) fat, sugar, and processed foods and to eat more fruits, vegetables, nuts, seeds, and other whole foods, limiting whole grains.

Overnutrition is many times worse than undernutrition. In fact, animal studies have shown that getting too few calories, which is technically called calorie restriction, can actually increase longevity.[6] Although I do recommend calorie restriction for some diseases, such as type 2 diabetes and obesity,[7] I believe that as a nation we need to work harder at eating in a way that keeps us within a healthy weight range.

Stop and Think About How You Eat

Our prosperity as a nation has come at a price. After years of overeating and overindulgence, we are experiencing an epidemic of degenerative diseases.

Most of us eat a standard American diet. That means lots of fat, sugar, and highly refined wheat and corn products, including white bread, crackers, bagels, pasta, and cereals. Add other processed food, such as potato chips, corn chips, and white rice. Don't forget the fatty meats such as T-bone steaks, ribs, bacon, and pork chops. Now top it all off with a large amount of saturated fat, hydrogenated fat, and polyunsaturated and processed vegetable fat, such as most salad dressings, most cooking oils, and mayonnaise. It's no wonder we have an epidemic of heart disease, cancer, diabetes, autoimmune disease, and arthritis, as well as many other degenerative and inflammatory diseases.

Now for dessert. What could be more American than apple pie? Nevertheless, the absolute worst foods—and all-time American favorites—contain tons of sugar and hydrogenated fat. These include many baked goods, such as cupcakes, cookies, pies, pastries, fudge, and brownies—and don't forget the doughnuts and candy bars.

We didn't always eat this way. Former generations were some of the healthiest on the planet. As part of an agrarian culture, many of our grandparents lived much closer to the land. But today our lifestyle is much too stressed and fast-paced, and as a result, our diet suffers.

CHANGE THE WAY YOU THINK

Most of us have grown up eating the American diet and feeling pretty good about it. But to live healthier, longer lives, we must rethink what we have been taught about food—before it's too late.

We begin to change our thinking by changing the why of eating. Just why do you eat? Do you eat because something tastes good and your flesh is craving it or because you are stressed, anxious, lonely, or depressed? Or do you eat because you are providing your body with fuel to run? For most Americans, eating has become more of a recreation than a daily necessity based upon nutritional wisdom.

Now I'm not trying to suggest that meals shouldn't be enjoyed. God created all things for us to enjoy, and eating was one of those things. But when our dietary choices, which were designed to nourish and sustain our bodies, actually begin to make us ill, then we must change the way we think.

Hippocrates, the father of medicine, is credited with saying, "Let thy food be thy medicine and thy medicine be thy food." In other words, what we eat should be so good for us that it actually heals and restores our bodies. What a difference from the average American mindset about eating!

Start thinking about more than just taste and pleasure when you eat. Begin to eat for your health's sake! Eventually you will enjoy and crave healthy foods like I do.

So here's your new set of priorities: health first, taste and pleasure second. I guarantee that once you begin to satisfy the true need of your body—the need for genuine nourishment—you will begin to enjoy your food much more.

Right now, before you even begin to follow my fasting program, determine that the minute the fast is over, you will start following a health-first eating lifestyle. Before you begin the fasting program, go through your cupboards, pantry, refrigerator, and freezer, and eliminate fried foods (chips, french fries, chicken nuggets, etc.), processed foods (any food that humans have tampered with and packaged, such as instant oatmeal, instant rice, most cereals, etc.), processed vegetable fats, saturated fats, hydrogenated and partially hydrogenated fats, and sugary foods.

Prepare a grocery list now for your new health-first eating plan, and stock your pantry in preparation for day twenty-nine. Keep plenty of organic extra-virgin olive oil and avocado oil. Determine to avoid fatty cuts of meats and to select smaller portions of the leanest meats, including free-range or organic chicken or turkey breast and free-range, grass-fed, organic beef such as extra-lean ground round, tenderloin, and filet.

USDA Guidelines

In your new health-first eating plan, you will want to eat at least five servings of living, organic vegetables and fruits every day. (By *living*, I mean that the naturally occurring nutrients in the plants have not been altered or depleted through processing, packaging, storage, or preparation.) In its *2015–2020 Dietary Guidelines for Americans*, the USDA recommends that fruits and vegetables make up half of your plate at every meal.[8] That means fruits and vegetables should comprise a large percentage of your diet. Fruits should be mainly organic berries, which are low glycemic.

Limit Meats

Most Americans eat far too much meat. I recommend that women eat only two to three ounces of lean, free-range meat once or twice daily. Men, limit meats to only three to six ounces of lean, free-range meat once or twice daily. And I always recommend chewing every bite twenty to thirty times.

Avoid High-Protein Diets

More and more people are going on high-protein diets such as the Atkins diet. Yes, they are losing weight. But the long-term effects of this diet can be very dangerous and may lead to many degenerative diseases.[9]

If you are on this diet, limit your protein portions to no more than three to six ounces for men and two to three ounces for women once or twice a day. Also, choose more monounsaturated fats such as olive oil, avocado oil, seeds, and nuts, and limit saturated and polyunsaturated fats.

IN CONCLUSION

If you see yourself in this chapter, be encouraged. Even if you have spent a lifetime digging your own grave with your fork and knife, it's never too late to change. You will make many choices about your destiny by what you choose to eat. Choose now to reap health, happiness, and a long life. You hold the key to your own future health.

Before we begin the fasting program, let's look at what I believe is the single most effective answer to overnourishment: fasting! More than anything else, fasting is a dynamic key to cleansing your body from a lifelong collection of toxins, reversing overnourishment and the diseases it brings, and ensuring a wonderful future of renewed energy, vitality, longevity, and blessed health.

CHAPTER 7

THE DETOX PLAN

THIS CHAPTER IS an introduction to my fasting program. It will provide you with the information you need to prepare for the actual fasting part of this detoxification and cleansing program. Before you consider fasting, it is important to follow this uniquely designed nutritional program to strengthen and support your liver, which will prepare it for the increased role of detoxification during your fast.

Your body was uniquely created to handle enormous amounts of toxins, poisons, germs, and free radicals. Your body's detoxification system, including your liver and GI tract, is astonishingly powerful. With proper nutritional support from you, it can both detoxify and eliminate chemicals and toxins.

A detoxification system that is functioning at peak efficiency has unending benefits for you, including these:

- prevents and even reverses disease

- provides you with more energy and mental clarity

- allows you to feel better

- aids you in losing weight

- helps clear up your skin and complexion

The first system of toxic cleansing is your liver. It's an amazing organ that works day and night to cleanse your blood from chemicals, poisons, bacteria, viruses, and any other foreign invaders that come to rob you of your good health. If your liver is not strong and healthy, you will not be strong and healthy. That's why it is so important for you to spend the first twenty-one days of my fasting program strengthening your liver so it can carry out its key role in the detoxification process.

If you wanted to be an Olympic award-winning athlete, you wouldn't enter the competition without spending months in training, strengthening your muscles, developing your skills, and building your body with the best diet and nutrition available. In the same way you must train your body to compete against the toxic world in which you live. The good news is that it's a competition you can win. But you have an enormous part in ensuring the long-term successful outcome.

Your Twenty-One-Day Liver-Support Program

For the first three weeks of my fasting program, you will follow this diet and regimen of supplements to prepare your body for fasting. It would even be very beneficial for you to restore your body following the fasting part of the program by repeating another one-week liver-support diet.

These dietary guidelines will help cleanse and support your liver while you fast and will continue helping your body to operate at peak efficiency as you begin your health-first lifestyle at the conclusion of my fasting program. The more closely you follow these guidelines, the more benefit you will receive from your fast. It is important that you change your diet and lifestyle to reduce the amount of toxins you are taking in as well as improve your body's ability to eliminate toxins.

This twenty-one-day fasting program will give you the necessary dietary guidelines to cleanse and support your liver. To get the optimum benefit, be careful to strictly follow these guidelines.

Foods to Avoid

Making the right choices of food for your liver's health is important, especially before you consider detoxification through fasting. Here are some foods (and other products) to avoid:

- colas and chocolate

- alcohol (including wine)

- processed vegetable oils

- animal skins and meats

- deep-fried foods

- microwaved foods

- hydrogenated and partially hydrogenated fats and oils, which are always found in most commercial peanut butter, margarine, and shortening but are also often included in foods such as bread, cake mixes, frozen foods, breakfast cereals, potato chips, and more (read all labels carefully)

- refined foods and processed foods, including white bread, chips, cereals, instant oatmeal, and instant rice
- simple sugars, including honey, syrup, agave, pastries, cookies, candies, cakes, and pies
- fast foods
- processed juices
- wheat products, including crackers, bagels, pasta, muffins
- corn products
- soy products
- dairy products, including butter, cheese, milk, yogurt, sour cream, and ice cream
- beans, peas, and lentils
- eggs
- fish and poultry
- nightshades (tomatoes, potatoes, paprika, eggplant, and peppers), since these foods are inflammatory for many with arthritis and autoimmune disease
- all grains, including wheat, corn, rice, barley, oats, and quinoa

For this detoxification fasting program, I have eliminated all meat, dairy, eggs, and other foods that commonly trigger allergic reactions or food sensitivity reactions, including corn, soy, wheat, and processed foods. Sprouted breads such as Ezekiel and manna bread are not allowed during this program because many people are sensitive to gluten. If you are allergic or sensitive to certain nuts, you will need to avoid those too.

FOODS TO EAT

For at least two weeks, in preparation for your fast, eat as many of the following foods as possible. Because certain fruits and vegetables have higher pesticide residues than others, especially the "Dirty Dozen," I strongly recommend organic for these. (To see the "Dirty Dozen" and "Clean Fifteen" lists from the Environmental Working Group, visit www.ewg.org/foodnews/.)

- Organic fruit: Berries including strawberries, blue-berries, raspberries, blackberries, and cranberries arc best for the liver. Drink a glass of freshly squeezed lemon or lime juice in the morning. (See appendix A for Green and Red Supremefood.)

- Organic vegetables: Eat as many raw or steamed veg-etables as possible. In addition, cruciferous vegeta-bles, such as cabbage, cauliflower, brussels sprouts, broccoli, kale, collard greens, mustard greens, and turnips, are very important. Other liver-friendly veg-etables include beets, carrots, dandelion root, water-cress, and greens—romaine lettuce, field greens, and arugula. You may steam the veggies or lightly stir-fry them in organic extra-virgin avocado, macadamia nut, or olive oil. (See appendix A for Green and Red Supremefood.)

- Good fats for your liver and for detoxification: Use organic, extra-virgin olive oil; avocados; raw, fresh nuts such as almonds, macadamia nuts, and walnuts (avoid peanuts and cashews); flaxseed oil (not for cooking); evening primrose oil; black currant seed oil; borage oil; and fish oil.

- Beverages: Drink plenty of pure, clean alkaline or spring water, with or without fresh-squeezed lemon or lime (two quarts daily), fresh vegetable and fruit juices, organic green tea or black tea, and other herbal teas. I recommend that you start drinking organic coffee or tea, and one cup of organic coffee per day is allowable, but use almond or coconut milk instead of creamer and stevia instead of sugar.

SUPPLEMENTS FOR THE LIVER

Because certain supplements are very important to the liver, you should take them when preparing for a detoxification fast and when ending a fast. For a complete discussion of important liver supplements, please see my book *Toxic Relief.* Following is a summary of the important supplements that I recommend you take every day of the first twenty-one days—the liver-support phase—of this fasting program. (Where indicated, see the appendix for the supplement's brand name.)

- a comprehensive multivitamin and mineral supplement (See appendix A.)

- milk thistle (200 ng two to three times a day, available at health food stores)

- N-acetylcysteine (NAC) or MaxOne

- organic green tea, dandelion tea, other herb teas (available at health food stores)

- phytonutrient powder/drink (See appendix A.)

- a soluble/insoluble fiber supplement (See appendix A.)

It Takes a Positive Attitude

The successful completion of this fasting program requires a winning attitude and the support of your friends and loved ones. To make necessary lifestyle changes, it is important that you not only have a determined attitude but also maintain a positive and cheerful outlook.

Discuss this part of the fasting program with your family. Whether or not they are joining you in this fast, it is best to discuss the program with them first. This would be an excellent time to sit down together as a family and create the guidelines for your new health-first lifestyle that you will launch at the end of the fast. Supportive family and friends working together and encouraging each other throughout the fasting program and on into your new lifestyle are a powerful force for success.

As you begin this phase, it is extremely important now for you to make the decision to eliminate toxins from your life. This should be a permanent decision for you, and it is essential during the fasting program. Avoid cigarette smoke, alcohol, and drugs. Decrease your intake of all medications. Of course, for prescription medicines, you must do this with your doctor's help. Be sensible; never make drastic changes without consulting your doctor.

OTHER TIPS AND TECHNIQUES

- Do not cut or prepare fruits and vegetables before you are ready to eat them. You may be tempted to slice up that melon and carrot just for the convenience of being able to grab them from the refrigerator, but fruits and vegetables lose their nutrients when they are cut and stored. It's best to prepare them when you know they will be immediately eaten.

- Don't deplete your food of nutrients by improper cooking techniques. When you boil vegetables, most of the nutrients leave the vegetables and end up in the water. By the time you eat them, the boiled water has a greater nutrient content than the vegetables themselves! (Soups, however, are an exception to this rule because you do consume the broth that contains the nutrients from the vegetables.) It's best to either steam veggies or eat them raw.

- If you must boil vegetables, bring the water to a boil first and then add your veggies to the water for a brief time. Do not allow them to soak in the water. Drain them immediately and serve them. I strongly recommend steaming your vegetables or eating them raw. I also recommend that my patients avoid microwaved foods altogether.

- Don't prepare too much food or prepare it too far ahead of time. Reheating food and leftovers depletes the food of valuable vitamins and other nutrients[1]— especially if you reheat in the microwave. A 1998 study found that just "six minutes of microwave cooking destroyed half of the vitamin B_{12} in dairy foods and meat, a much higher rate of destruction than other cooking techniques."[2]

- Fruits and vegetables should be eaten unpeeled whenever possible because many vitamins and minerals are actually concentrated in or just beneath their skin. If you have not purchased organic items, it is imperative that you wash these fruits and vegetables carefully to remove pesticides.

- It is best to use fresh, organically grown produce. However, if fresh products are not available, choose frozen fruits and vegetables. Only rarely should you choose canned fruits and vegetables, making sure the label lists only organic, whole ingredients.

BEFORE YOU BEGIN

Before you start, it's important to set the boundaries of your fast. Determine what type of fast you will go on. Check the boxes below that identify the fast or fasts you will be implementing.

- ❏ a partial fast to support the liver during detoxification
- ❏ a Daniel fast, as in the Book of Daniel
- ❏ a fruit and vegetable juice fast

One final note: As you look through the daily meal plans, keep in mind that these are only suggestions provided to give you variety. All the recipes are provided in appendix B and are grouped into three categories: smoothies, salads, and soups. This will allow you to substitute, combine, and/or repeat any meal according to your tastes. I do ask that you limit yourself to the recipes given in this book and that you follow the recipes exactly as written to ensure that you receive the benefits of detoxifying your body. If you want, you can choose to substitute vegetable and fruit juices for some of the meal suggestions. There are some juice recipes in appendix B as well.

You can also sign up for my 21 Day Detox program online at www.DivineHealthDetox.com. Sign-up is free and includes videos of helpful instruction and a printable detox shopping list.

My hope is that these days of cleansing and healing will be some of the most rewarding days of your entire life. I am confident that you will experience renewed health, energy, and vitality!

Now it's time to get started.

The Detox Meal Plan

DAY 1

MEAL SUGGESTIONS

Breakfast: Blueberry Smoothie
Lunch: Dr. C's Chopped Salad
Dinner: Fasting Zone Hot and Sour Soup

FOCUS THOUGHT

Without a healthy, well-functioning liver and a healthy intestinal tract, your body will continue to labor under a dangerous burden of toxins.

YOUR DAILY PRESCRIPTION FOR HEALTH

With a special diet to get your liver and GI tract in shape and a program of short, easy juice fasts, together with some lifestyle changes, you really can cleanse your body. By cleansing your system of built-up toxins, you truly will feel better than you have in years. Deep cleansing your body right down to the cellular level will renew your vitality, restore your energy, reclaim your health, shed toxic fat, lengthen your life, and give you a healthy glow.

RECORD YOUR THOUGHTS

Take time to record your thoughts and experiences as you fast.

DAY 2

MEAL SUGGESTIONS

Breakfast: Raspberry Smoothie
Lunch: Strawberry Spinach Salad
Dinner: Artichoke and Mushroom Soup

FOCUS THOUGHT

It is important to understand that your thinking patterns and emotional responses affect your body. God desires for you to be totally well, physically, mentally, emotionally, and spiritually.

YOUR DAILY PRESCRIPTION FOR HEALTH

Fasting provides your body, mind, and spirit with many benefits. Medical science is recognizing more and more the innate connection between these inseparable facets of our being. What we eat affects our moods and, to a certain extent, even our attitudes. What we think affects how our bodies digest food and impacts the way we handle stress. And our spiritual well-being is influenced by our physical and mental health.

Toxic emotions such as anger, resentment, fear, anxiety, grief, and depression can create excessive stress, whereas positive emotions such as gratitude, joy, love, and peace actually relieve stress. The physical effects of reprogramming your thoughts begin with your heart. Your heartbeat varies from moment to moment based on your emotions and attitudes.[3]

When you experience stress and negative emotions such as anger, frustration, fear, and anxiety, your heart rate variability pattern becomes "more erratic and disordered," and it sends chaotic signals to the brain. The result is energy drain and "added wear and tear" on your mind and body. "In contrast, sustained positive emotions, such as appreciation, love, and compassion, are associated with highly ordered...patterns in the heart rhythms" and a significant reduction of stress.[4]

RECORD YOUR THOUGHTS

Take time to record your thoughts and experiences as you fast.

DAY 3

MEAL SUGGESTIONS

Breakfast: Strawberry Smoothie
Lunch: Kale and Veggie Salad
Dinner: Veggie Soup With Avocado

FOCUS THOUGHT

Forgiveness enables the body to release toxins. Choose to extend forgiveness today—this includes forgiving yourself.

YOUR DAILY PRESCRIPTION FOR HEALTH

Many individuals rehash, relive, and meditate on painful experiences of their past. They relive the hurt over and over, and they never heal. These individuals are harboring an offense—a circumstance that is perceived as unjust or hurtful.

When you harbor an offense, you usually deal with the problem by thinking and talking about it too much. The sad thing is that holding unforgiveness in your heart literally locks toxins inside your body.

When you fail to forgive, you stimulate the stress response in your body. This causes chronic stimulation of the sympathetic nervous system and elevation of stress hormones, which in turn causes constriction of blood vessels and locks toxins in the body. For more information on this topic, please refer to my book *Deadly Emotions.*[5]

RECORD YOUR THOUGHTS

Take time to record your thoughts and experiences as you fast.

DAY 4

MEAL SUGGESTIONS

Breakfast: Blackberry Smoothie
Lunch: Fasting Zone Cole Slaw
Dinner: Garden Veggie Detox Soup

FOCUS THOUGHT

Let what you take into your body provide healing. "Let thy medicine be thy food and thy food be thy medicine" (frequently credited to Hippocrates).

YOUR DAILY PRESCRIPTION FOR HEALTH

Fasting is good for you on so many levels. Few things you can do for your body have as much power as fasting does to radically improve your physical health. Fasting helps to break food addictions and other unhealthy eating habits.

After a fast, fresh fruits and vegetables taste wonderful. And you won't desire to binge or overeat as you receive the nourishment your body needs.

So don't be alarmed. Fasting doesn't have to be scary. It will improve your health physically and spiritually.

RECORD YOUR THOUGHTS

Take time to record your thoughts and experiences as you fast.

DAY 5

MEAL SUGGESTIONS

Breakfast: Lemon Smoothie

Lunch: Arugula and Asparagus Salad

Dinner: Detoxifying Cabbage Soup

FOCUS THOUGHT

You can wean yourself from unhealthy eating habits by consciously substituting "dead food" products that have been your old favorites with "living foods." For example, choose a large Greek salad with extra-virgin olive oil instead of choosing a burger, fries, and a soda.

YOUR DAILY PRESCRIPTION FOR HEALTH

Living foods—organic fruits, vegetables, nuts, and seeds—produce life. Human-made food is generally "dead," meaning it has no enzymes and will usually be deficient in vitamins, minerals, antioxidants, and phytonutrients. Dead foods include most fast foods, sugary foods, processed foods, junk foods, and snack foods. Excessive intake of dead foods eventually leads to degenerative diseases and early death.[6]

RECORD YOUR THOUGHTS

Take time to record your thoughts and experiences as you fast.

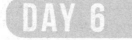

DAY 6

MEAL SUGGESTIONS

Breakfast: Lime Smoothie
Lunch: Watercress and Avocado Salad
Dinner: Creamy Carrot and Coconut Soup

FOCUS THOUGHT

Humble fasting before God is awesomely powerful and can turn an entire nation around.

YOUR DAILY PRESCRIPTION FOR HEALTH

Choosing your foods is the first step toward a health-first lifestyle, but the way you prepare those foods is just as important. Deep-frying causes food (french fries, chicken, chicken strips, onion rings, etc.) to soak up free radicals and lose nutrients. There are much healthier ways to cook your food. Stir-frying is a good method since the food is cooked so briefly that it retains most of its nutrients.

Simply use a moderate amount of avocado or macadamia nut oil. Grilling is also generally safe. Use a propane gas grill in place of charcoal or mesquite, which contain dangerous toxins. Place the vegetable or meat rack as high as possible away from the flame.

If meat cooks over a flame, the fat drips off the meat and into the fire, which turns it into steam. The pesticides in the fat char into the meat so that even greater amounts of carcinogens are formed. Avoid charring meat since the charring contains a chemical called benzopyrene, which is a highly carcinogenic substance.[7] Scrape or cut off the char.

RECORD YOUR THOUGHTS

Take time to record your thoughts and experiences as you fast.

DAY 7

MEAL SUGGESTIONS

Breakfast: Cherry Smoothie
Lunch: Strawberry Spinach Salad
Dinner: Veggie Soup With Avocado

FOCUS THOUGHT

Tap water may contain heavy metals, pesticides, bacteria, other microbes, chlorine, fluoride, aluminum, and many other chemicals and toxins. It's best not to drink tap water or use it for cooking.

YOUR DAILY PRESCRIPTION FOR HEALTH

Many people choose to drink tap water; however, this is not a wise choice. According to the Environmental Working Group (EWG), tests of drinking water throughout America found 267 contaminants that brought an increased risk of all kinds of medical conditions, including cancer.[8] However, the EPA currently regulates only ninety contaminants.[9] Municipal treatment plants cannot remove most chemicals from the water supply.[10] The underground aquifers that feed city water supplies may catch runoff from dump sites, landfills, and even underground storage tanks.

Sooner or later anything we bury, spray, emit, or flush finds its way into our drinking water. Tap water is good for watering lawns, washing clothes, and flushing toilets, but not for drinking or cooking. If you have been drinking tap water or beverages made from tap water (iced tea, coffee, etc.), I strongly recommend that you purchase either a water filter or pure, bottled water. For more information on this topic, refer to my book *The Seven Pillars of Health*.[11]

RECORD YOUR THOUGHTS

Take time to record your thoughts and experiences as you fast.

DAY 8

MEAL SUGGESTIONS

Breakfast: Blueberry Smoothie
Lunch: Kale and Veggie Salad
Dinner: Garden Veggie Detox Soup

FOCUS THOUGHT

When you sit down to eat, take time to thank God and to meditate on all His goodness and provision. Release any negative emotions, bless the food, and then begin to eat.

YOUR DAILY PRESCRIPTION FOR HEALTH

Make dining your most pleasant times of the day—especially dinner. It should be a time to slow down, relax, and gather with family and friends to enjoy the food and fellowship. The atmosphere at mealtime should be peaceful, pleasant, and joyful. Turn off the television; don't even watch sporting events, the news, or movies. Begin your meal with a blessing, and then pause and consider how thankful you are. Always keep the conversation pleasant, and never use the dinner table as a time to reprimand your children or discuss stressful topics for yourself or your children. Never argue or complain at the table, but instead choose to compliment, encourage, tell funny or entertaining stories, and simply relax and fellowship with one another.

At restaurants I commonly hear families arguing, complaining, and fussing with one another. Realize that when you are stressed, you can't digest as well and are more prone to develop heartburn, indigestion, bloating, and gas.

If you are angry, upset, or just irritated, then wait to eat. When families sit down to a meal together, especially dinner, parents are given a chance to reconnect with their children.

Make it a point to create a pleasant environment at mealtime, and if arguments or complaints begin, redirect the conversation to wholesome, pleasant topics.

RECORD YOUR THOUGHTS

Take time to record your thoughts and experiences as you fast.

DAY 9

MEAL SUGGESTIONS

Breakfast: Raspberry Smoothie
Lunch: Fasting Zone Cole Slaw
Dinner: Detoxifying Cabbage Soup

FOCUS THOUGHT

Don't overeat. Eat only until you are satisfied and no more. Overeating places an enormous added burden on your liver and detoxification pathways.

YOUR DAILY PRESCRIPTION FOR HEALTH

The main reason many Americans are obese is simply gluttony. Interestingly, a study from Purdue University found that religious people are more likely to be overweight than are nonreligious people.[12]

If you tend to be an overeater, here are some pointers that can help. Fill your plate in the kitchen and place it on the table rather than serving yourself at the table. Chew your food slowly (each bite should be chewed twenty to thirty times), and rest between bites. Set your fork down between bites. Give your stomach a chance to find out how full it is before you give it more.

It generally takes twenty minutes for the brain to inform you that you are full or satisfied, so slow down while eating. A deep breath at the end of a meal is generally a sign that your body is satisfied. Plan a walk right after dinner. When you dine out, take half your order home for the next day or split the meal with your spouse.

RECORD YOUR THOUGHTS

Take time to record your thoughts and experiences as you fast.

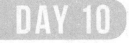

DAY 10

MEAL SUGGESTIONS

Breakfast: Strawberry Smoothie
Lunch: Arugula and Asparagus Salad
Dinner: Creamy Carrot and Coconut Soup

FOCUS THOUGHT

You are what you eat—especially when it comes to your physical body. And what you eat will make all the difference in maintaining, strengthening, and detoxifying your liver.

YOUR DAILY PRESCRIPTION FOR HEALTH

Everything you put in your mouth has the potential to produce life or death. Consistently eating the wrong foods will eventually cause poor health and disease.

All foods are not created equal. Living foods were created for our consumption. They exist in a raw or close-to-raw state. Living foods include fruit, vegetables, seeds, and nuts. No chemicals have been added. They have not been bleached or chemically altered. Living foods are plucked, harvested, and squeezed, not processed, packaged, and put on a shelf.

If you want to be healthy, vibrant, and energetic, then you must begin to choose to eat more living foods. If you can eat at least 50 percent of your food as living food, you are much more likely to be healthy and resistant to most diseases.

RECORD YOUR THOUGHTS

Take time to record your thoughts and experiences as you fast.

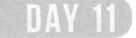

MEAL SUGGESTIONS

Breakfast: Blackberry Smoothie
Lunch: Watercress and Avocado Salad
Dinner: Fasting Zone Hot and Sour Soup

FOCUS THOUGHT

Wisdom is a pathway that God has given us to walk upon.
When we choose to walk in wisdom, the benefits to our
lives and health are limitless.

YOUR DAILY PRESCRIPTION FOR HEALTH

As an antioxidant, green tea is twenty-five times more powerful than vitamin E and one hundred times more powerful
than vitamin C.[13] Green tea is believed to block the effect of

cancer-causing chemicals. It also activates detoxification enzymes in the liver, which helps defend your body against cancer.[14] For detoxification purposes I recommend one cup of organic green tea two to three times a day. If you prefer, you may take green tea in capsule form.

As you can imagine by now, antioxidants are extremely important in this vital work of your liver. Glutathione is one of the most important and abundant antioxidants in the body. The liver is a hotbed of free-radical activity, and adequate levels of glutathione are essential to prevent damage by free radicals. The amino acid N-acetyl-cysteine (NAC) is converted in the body to glutathione.

In my opinion glutathione is the most important antioxidant in the body and is very important for detoxification. For more information on glutathione refer to my book *Toxic Relief.*

RECORD YOUR THOUGHTS

Take time to record your thoughts and experiences as you fast.

DAY 12

MEAL SUGGESTIONS

Breakfast: Lemon Smoothie
Lunch: Dr. C's Chopped Salad
Dinner: Artichoke and Mushroom Soup

FOCUS THOUGHT

If you want an easy, natural way to boost your self-image, build your confidence, and increase your energy, determine to exercise at least twenty minutes a day, three to four days a week.

YOUR DAILY PRESCRIPTION FOR HEALTH

I recommend that to ensure a healthy, fasted lifestyle, you plan to include a good exercise program. Many toxins can be expelled simply through perspiration as you give your body the exercise it needs. Exercise is also an antidote for stress, helping to relax tight muscles and release the tension of the day.

Regular exercise improves heart health, lung function, circulation, and blood pressure. Exercise can actually decrease fatigue as it relaxes your muscles and reduces stress. As you exercise, your body also releases endorphins, which are natural antide-pressants and pain relievers, that results in your feeling better after you exercise.

Aerobic exercise helps to calm your body as well as your mind by releasing tension. During your fast it is best to keep this exercise light so that you do not become overly tired. You may want to get together with friends for a walk, tennis, or a bike ride. Choose to exercise in a way that is enjoyable to you, and you will be more likely to succeed in it.

RECORD YOUR THOUGHTS

Take time to record your thoughts and experiences as you fast.

DAY 13

MEAL SUGGESTIONS

Breakfast: Lime Smoothie
Lunch: Kale and Veggie Salad
Dinner: Detoxifying Cabbage Soup

FOCUS THOUGHT

Don't eat when you're stressed. Before you pick up your
fork, take a brief moment to relax a bit by taking five to
ten slow, deep abdominal breaths. It's extremely important.

YOUR DAILY PRESCRIPTION FOR HEALTH

The efficiency of your GI tract is being challenged every day.
One of those challenges comes from a deficiency of the incredibly powerful digestive juices. If you are over fifty years old, you
may be among the many middle-aged individuals who begin to
experience a reduction in the hydrochloric acid and pancreatic
enzymes that are so essential to digestion. When the levels of
this acid become depleted, digestive problems follow.

If stress plays a major role in your life, you probably don't
need me to tell you that it affects digestion. It's not unusual for
stressed-out individuals to have stomach medications strewed all
around their workplace and home. If you are stressed, you are
probably deficient in not only hydrochloric acid but usually pancreatic enzymes as well.

The lack of these vital pancreatic enzymes causes poor

digestion of proteins, fats, and carbohydrates. When this happens, bits of partially digested food can putrefy and eventually may lead to bacterial overgrowth in the small intestines, food sensitivities, leaky gut (increased intestinal permeability), irritable bowel syndrome, and so forth.[15]

RECORD YOUR THOUGHTS

Take time to record your thoughts and experiences as you fast.

DAY 14

MEAL SUGGESTIONS

Breakfast: Cherry Smoothie
Lunch: Fasting Zone Cole Slaw
Dinner: Creamy Carrot and Coconut Soup

FOCUS THOUGHT

If poor lifestyle choices have brought disease into your body, don't condemn yourself; God does not condemn you. Begin making better choices based upon godly wisdom.

YOUR DAILY PRESCRIPTION FOR HEALTH

Fiber is fantastic for your healthy GI tract. It acts like a broom, sweeping the colon lining, eliminating the toxins, and binding toxins and bile so that they cannot be reabsorbed back into your body. All of this activity is critically important in preventing disease. High-fiber diets also reduce the level of circulating estrogens by binding them and preventing them from being reabsorbed and recirculated through the liver.[16]

Most of the chemicals that have been detoxified by the liver are contained in the bile, which is then dumped into the intestinal tract. This, as you know, is a major part of your body's detoxification process. But if your GI tract doesn't have enough fiber or is constipated, then much of that toxic bile will be reabsorbed back into your body.[17]

That's why it's so important to get plenty of fiber every day through your diet and to supplement with fiber regularly as well so that the toxins in your body will be bound and excreted. This will dramatically reduce your body's toxic burden.

RECORD YOUR THOUGHTS

Take time to record your thoughts and experiences as you fast.

DAY 15

MEAL SUGGESTIONS

Breakfast: Blueberry Smoothie
Lunch: Arugula and Asparagus Salad
Dinner: Fasting Zone Hot and Sour Soup

FOCUS THOUGHT

Digestion actually begins when your brain signals that your body needs food. When you start thinking about the minestrone you are making for dinner, your brain signals your digestive tract to begin producing the necessary enzymes and components for digestion.

YOUR DAILY PRESCRIPTION FOR HEALTH

Imagine that your skin suddenly turned to glass so that you could see everything going on inside you. You would quickly see that your intestinal tract is, stated simply, a long, winding tube. As a matter of fact, it is a continuous tube that averages about twenty feet long.[18] It connects your entire digestive system together. Your food enters the tube on one end and exits on the other.

In between, your food undergoes a miracle of processing. The mouth starts the process and connects with the esophagus. The esophagus connects with the stomach. The stomach connects with the small intestines. The small intestines connect with the large intestines, and the large intestines connect to the rectum

and finally end at the anus. If digestion and elimination pro-
ceed smoothly and unhindered and you consume enough water
and fiber, then toxins are eliminated daily, and good health is
achieved.

RECORD YOUR THOUGHTS

Take time to record your thoughts and experiences as you fast.

DAY 16

MEAL SUGGESTIONS

Breakfast: Raspberry Smoothie
Lunch: Watercress and Avocado Salad
Dinner: Artichoke and Mushroom Soup

FOCUS THOUGHT

When you go on a water-only fast, mechanisms in your brain eventually signal your body that you are starving even if you are not. Therefore, your body goes into a survival state to try and hold on to all the calories it gets.

YOUR DAILY PRESCRIPTION FOR HEALTH

The strictest, most severe fast is a water-only fast. In general I usually don't recommend this type of fasting. But for certain autoimmune diseases such as lupus and rheumatoid arthritis or for severe atherosclerosis such as severe coronary artery disease, the benefits of water-only fasting are powerful in select individuals.

Nevertheless, you can also experience similar benefits for these diseases with juice fasting—it just takes longer. For most individuals, water-only fasting so weakens the body that working a full-time job while fasting is not usually possible. Juice fasting provides most of the benefits of water-only fasting without the unpleasant weakness and hunger that often accompany a water-only fast.

RECORD YOUR THOUGHTS

Take time to record your thoughts and experiences as you fast.

DAY 17

MEAL SUGGESTIONS

Breakfast: Strawberry Smoothie
Lunch: Dr. C's Chopped Salad
Dinner: Veggie Soup With Avocado

FOCUS THOUGHT

Isn't it interesting that God placed beautiful colors of red, blue, and purple in different fruits and vegetables that provide protection from most diseases and actually keep you looking younger?

YOUR DAILY PRESCRIPTION FOR HEALTH

Flavonoids are a group of powerful phytonutrients. A type of flavonoids called anthocyanins are primarily found in red, purple, and blue plant pigments, especially blackberries, blueberries, cherries, and grapes.[19] Flavonoids can keep your skin looking younger because they play an enormous role in the formation and repair of collagen.[20]

Collagen is both the primary structural protein and the most abundant protein found in your body. It actually holds the cells and tissues of your body together. Collagen tends to degenerate with age and slowly collapse, which is why our skin begins to wrinkle and sag as we get older. However, the flavonoids found in berries, cherries, grapes, and a host of other fruits and vegetables help to maintain the integrity of your skin's collagen.

Therefore, it helps to keep your skin's collagen from degenerating and collapsing with age. By simply juicing berries every day, you can get enough flavonoids to nourish your skin's collagen and slow down the aging process.

RECORD YOUR THOUGHTS

Take time to record your thoughts and experiences as you fast.

DAY 18

MEAL SUGGESTIONS

Breakfast: Blackberry Smoothie
Lunch: Strawberry Spinach Salad
Dinner: Garden Veggie Detox Soup

FOCUS THOUGHT

Are you listening to your body? Do you understand what it is trying to tell you? How is your physical body responding to my fasting program?

YOUR DAILY PRESCRIPTION FOR HEALTH

The main causes of increased intestinal permeability (microscopic openings or holes in the small intestine caused by inflammation) are food allergies, food sensitivities, and, many times, antibiotic usage. Common food allergies include allergies to egg, dairy products, corn, soy, yeast, wheat, and other grains such as rye, barley, and oats. The main protein that people are sensitive to in these grains is gluten, which is found in breads, crackers, pasta, all kinds of flour (such as rye, barley, wheat and oat flour), gravies, many soups, bread crumbs, pies, and cakes.

Increased intestinal permeability is usually present in the following diseases: chronic fatigue, fibromyalgia, Crohn's disease, ulcerative colitis, celiac disease, rheumatoid arthritis, lupus,[21] migraine headaches, eczema, hives, psoriasis,[22] schizophrenia, autism, and attention-deficit hyperactivity disorder.[23]

If you suspect this might be an issue for you, this liver detoxification and fasting program should benefit you. If you are sensitive to gluten, select another form of grain for your daily diet, such as brown rice bread, millet bread, quinoa, kamut, or amaranth. Buckwheat is also gluten-free, so you can still have buckwheat pancakes. However, it is best to avoid all grains while on the Detox Meal Plan.

RECORD YOUR THOUGHTS

Take time to record your thoughts and experiences as you fast.

DAY 19

MEAL SUGGESTIONS

Breakfast: Lemon Smoothie
Lunch: Fasting Zone Cole Slaw
Dinner: Artichoke and Mushroom Soup

FOCUS THOUGHT

Each lifestyle choice that you and I make leads us down a
pathway—to peace and joy or to stress and hardship. Be
sure you know where your choices are leading you.

YOUR DAILY PRESCRIPTION FOR HEALTH

Milk thistle extract, known as silymarin, is one of the most powerful protectors of the liver against free-radical damage. It also

protects the liver from many different extremely toxic chemicals, including the poisonous mushroom *Amanita phalloides*,[24] which is fatal in 10 to 20 percent of the people who ingest it.[25]

Vast amounts of the powerful antioxidant glutathione can be expended in the detoxification process, which can lead to glutathione depletion. Milk thistle will prevent this depletion during detoxification. Milk thistle can actually raise the level of glutathione in the liver up to 35 percent.[26] Milk thistle is one of the most important antioxidants to take during the detoxification fasting program.

RECORD YOUR THOUGHTS

Take time to record your thoughts and experiences as you fast.

DAY 20

MEAL SUGGESTIONS

Breakfast: Lime Smoothie
Lunch: Arugula and Asparagus Salad
Dinner: Veggie Soup With Avocado

FOCUS THOUGHT

If you take over-the-counter medicines, consider more natural ways to treat your various medical conditions, such as nutrients, herbs, and homeopathic medicines. However, you should never stop taking medications that you need without consulting your doctor.

YOUR DAILY PRESCRIPTION FOR HEALTH

Few people ever consider that the health of their bodies is based upon a delicate natural acid and alkaline balance. Nevertheless, this balance is essential to your body's ability to detoxify successfully. Veggies are crucial for helping you maintain a healthy pH.

When all your body gets is the standard American diet, your tissues become more acidic than nature intended, which upsets this delicate balance. If you would like to know how acidic your body is, you can find out very easily by simply purchasing some pH strips at the drugstore or health food store.

Collect the first morning urine, and dip a pH strip into it. The strip will indicate your urine's pH level with a change of color. The pH strip package includes a card that correlates each possible color with a pH number. Match the color of your pH strip to its numerical reading on the card.

The urinary pH usually indicates the pH of the tissues. Most people will have a pH test reading of about 5.0, which means their bodies are very acidic. It should be between 6.8 and 7.0. Close enough doesn't count. Even though 5 is only two points less than 7, a pH of 5.0 is actually a hundred times more acidic than a pH of 7.0.

A healthy stomach has a pH between 1.5 and 3.0 due to hydrochloric acid, which is secreted by the stomach. Hydrochloric acid is strong enough to burn a hole through the carpet or to melt the iron in a nail. You can see how this powerful acid forms the first line of defense against bacteria, parasites, germs, and other microbes from our food.

RECORD YOUR THOUGHTS

Take time to record your thoughts and experiences as you fast.

DAY 21

MEAL SUGGESTIONS

Breakfast: Cherry Smoothie
Lunch: Watercress and Avocado Salad
Dinner: Garden Veggie Detox Soup

FOCUS THOUGHT

Your amazing body is designed not only to detoxify itself
but also to heal itself. And just as you can play a significant
role in helping and supporting your body's own ability to
detoxify itself, you can also do the same with healing.

YOUR DAILY PRESCRIPTION FOR HEALTH

The most important nutrients in fresh fruits and juices are the
phytonutrients. Phytonutrients are simply plant-derived nutrients that contain powerful antioxidants and give fruits and vegetables their brilliant colors. These mighty plant nutrients prevent
tumors and cancer, lower cholesterol, increase immune function,
fight viruses, stimulate detoxification enzymes, prevent plaque
buildup (which protects us against heart disease), and block the
production of cancer-causing compounds.

Many of these phytonutrients are found in the pigments of the
fruits and vegetables, such as the chlorophyll of green vegetables,

the carotenes or carotenoids in orange fruits and vegetables, and the purple flavonoids in berries. One out of three Americans will at some time develop cancer in his or her lifetime.[27] Consuming adequate amounts of fruits and vegetables every day or in the form of juices is one of the best ways to protect your body from cancer and heart disease.

RECORD YOUR THOUGHTS

Take time to record your thoughts and experiences as you fast.

CHAPTER 8

LIFE AFTER DETOX

Y OU HAVE COME to the very important phase of breaking your fast. This is often the most difficult and most important part of fasting. Therefore, you must understand how to break your fast before you even begin.

Reintroduce foods gradually to realize the greatest health benefits of fasting. Your digestive tract has been at rest. That means hydrochloric acid and pancreatic enzymes may not be available to help you digest proteins, starches, and fats right away. Therefore, the longer your fast time, the more slowly you should come off your fast.

Some individuals who have not broken their fast properly have developed gallstones and have needed surgery. I gradually reintroduce fruit, then vegetables, then starches such as breads, and finally proteins and fats. Some may find it beneficial to take one to two tablespoons of lecithin granules (in two ounces of water) once or twice daily to prevent sludge in the gallbladder during this stage of the program.

Follow this four-day phase of breaking your fast to ensure the good health you have begun to achieve through the first two phases of my fasting program. If this was your first experience with a detoxifying fast, or if you suffer from poor health or numerous diseases, at the end of the four days you may repeat the twenty-one-day liver-support phase of my fasting program before you move on to the health-first lifestyle described in many of my books.

Your journey to good health is not over when the next four days have ended. Your journey is just beginning. Be ready to step into your new health-first lifestyle plan with these first four days after your fast.

The First Day After Your Detox

The first day after your fast, eat fresh fruit such as apples, watermelon, grapes, or fresh berries as often as every two to three hours. However, don't eat papaya or pineapple on the first day after a fast. These fruits contain strong enzymes that may upset your stomach. Fruits with the highest water content, such as watermelon, are the easiest to digest.

Have you prepared your shopping list to begin your new health-first lifestyle? Begin your shopping list today. When you go to the grocery store, shop for the following organic fruits and vegetables: carrots, cabbage, apples, cucumbers, beets, celery, parsley, berries (including strawberries, blackberries, blueberries, raspberries), lemons and limes, grapefruit, pineapple, ginger root, watermelon, garlic, greens (including spinach, collard greens, beet greens, dandelion greens), sweet potatoes, and dandelion root.

Meal suggestions

Breakfast

> fruit smoothie
>
> 1 scoop phytonutrient powder (optional; see appendix A)
>
> 1 teaspoon (level or heaping) psyllium husk powder or keto fiber in 4 ounces water

Lunch

> salad or soup with 1–2 ounces organic, pastured chicken

Evening Meal

> salad, soup, or smoothie
>
> 1 teaspoon (level or heaping) psyllium husk powder or keto fiber in 4 ounces water

Daily Supplements

> a multivitamin daily (see appendix A)
>
> a scoop of phytonutrient powder (see appendix A)

THE SECOND DAY AFTER YOUR DETOX

On the second day after you break your fast, have a fruit smoothie in the morning. For lunch and dinner have a bowl of fresh vegetable soup or a salad with 2–3 ounces of organic, pastured chicken or turkey; organic, grass-fed beef; or wild fish. Eat slowly, and chew your food very well. Be sure not to overeat. Be sure you continue to drink at least two quarts of clean, pure water a day. You may also continue to drink your juices once or twice a day.

Meal suggestions

Breakfast

> fruit smoothie
> 1 teaspoon (level or heaping) psyllium husk pow-
>   der or keto fiber in 4 ounces water

Lunch

> soup or salad with 2–3 ounces of wild fish

Evening Meal

> soup, salad, or smoothie
> 1 teaspoon (level or heaping) psyllium husk pow-
>   der or keto fiber in 4 ounces water

Daily Supplements

> a multivitamin daily (see appendix A)
> a scoop of phytonutrient powder (see appendix
>   A)

THE THIRD DAY AFTER YOUR DETOX

On the third day have a fruit smoothie in the morning. For lunch and dinner have a bowl of fresh vegetable soup or a salad with 2–3 ounces of organic, pastured chicken or turkey; organic, grass-fed beef; or wild fish. You may also add a baked potato or a slice of whole-grain bread such as Ezekiel or manna bread, brown rice bread, or millet bread.

Meal suggestions

Breakfast

> fruit smoothie
>
> 1 teaspoon (level or heaping) psyllium husk powder or keto fiber in 4 ounces water

Lunch

> soup or salad with 2–3 ounces of organic, pastured turkey

Dinner

> 1 bowl fresh vegetable soup
>
> 1 spinach salad or romaine salad with organic extra-virgin olive oil and apple cider vinegar
>
> 2–3 ounces of protein (chicken, turkey, beef, or fish)
>
> 1 teaspoon (level or heaping) psyllium husk powder or keto fiber in 4 ounces water

Daily Supplements

> a multivitamin daily (see appendix A)
>
> a scoop of phytonutrient powder (see appendix A)

The Fourth Day After Your Detox

On the fourth day continue with smoothies, soups, or salads with some healthy protein. I recommend that you try one of the following healthy methods for preparing your foods.

- Lightly steaming your vegetables causes very little loss of nutrients.

- Stir-frying is a good method of cooking because the food is briefly cooked and therefore retains most of its nutrients.

- Grilling is an acceptable means of food preparation. When grilling your free-range or organic meats, simply avoid charring the meat.

Meal suggestions

Breakfast

¼–½ cup berries

1–2 eggs cooked in avocado oil, topped with avocado slices

1 scoop phytonutrient powder (optional; see appendix A)

1 teaspoon (level or heaping) psyllium husk powder or keto fiber in 4 ounces water

Lunch

1 fresh vegetable salad

2–3 ounces grilled chicken breast

Dinner

1 cup fresh vegetable soup

1 small vegetable salad

2–3 ounces organic, pastured chicken or turkey; organic, grass-fed beef; or wild fish

1 teaspoon (level or heaping) psyllium husk powder or keto fiber in 4 ounces water

CHAPTER 9

INTERMITTENT FASTING

WHAT EXACTLY IS intermittent fasting? In the briefest of terms, intermittent fasting is going without food for a short amount of time.

You may have already done this by accident. Perhaps a pressure-filled work project or unexpected travel plans messed up your daily schedule and you ended up not eating for longer than was your usual pattern.

Many people eat until they go to bed and again as soon as they wake up. The six to eight hours of sleep is not enough time for your body to count it as fasting.

If the window of time where you don't eat is long enough, your body will think you are fasting! It doesn't have to be twenty-four hours, three days, three weeks, or even thirty days for your body to gain the benefits of fasting.

That is where intermittent fasting comes into play. There are quite a few different versions of intermittent fasting these days.

Patients coming through my offices may have tried all of them, including these popular methods:

- 12/12 plan: Eat during twelve hours of your day, and fast for twelve hours.

- 16/8 plan: Eat during eight hours of your day, and fast for sixteen hours. (This is my favorite.)

- 4/20 plan: Eat during four hours of your day, and fast for twenty hours.

- 5/2 plan (also called the 5:2 diet): Reduce your food intake to around five hundred calories twice a week, on two nonconsecutive days.

- Alternate-day plan: Eat no food for one day, eat normally the next day, fast again, eat again, and so on.

With all these intermittent fasting options, it is assumed that you will eat regular (and hopefully healthy!) food during the nonfasting times. And it is assumed that you will drink at least two quarts of clean, pure alkaline water during your fasting times. Staying hydrated is vitally important. You can also drink coffee, tea, or other select beverages as long as they contain no calories.

IT'S A FACT

Intermittent fasting can help lower blood pressure, thereby reducing the amount of needed blood pressure medication with its terrible side effects (brain fog, fatigue, erectile dysfunction, sluggishness, etc.). Intermittent fasting has helped hundreds of my patients with their blood pressure issues.

Also, it is assumed that a good portion of the time that you are not eating is spent sleeping. For example, in the common 16/8 plan, people fast for sixteen hours. If they sleep for eight hours, that means the eight additional waking hours are spent without food.

They might eat dinner at 5:00 p.m., finishing by 5:30 p.m. Then they might not eat breakfast until 9:30 the next morning. (If they want it, they can still have their coffee when they wake up.)

Or they might simply skip breakfast or dinner to help them attain the sixteen hours without food. This two-meal-a-day option reduces caloric intake considerably, which some people prefer to do and is my favorite.

One of my patients had lost weight with my Keto Zone diet, but she felt she had plateaued with her weight-loss plans. She started to fast sixteen hours a day, skipping breakfast, and it helped her body burn off additional fat. Those extra few hours of fasting gave her the benefits she was seeking.

Of all the intermittent fasting plans, schedules, and options, my preference is the 16/8 plan. Why? Because it works well with my patients' schedules, which increases the likelihood that they will keep doing it.

And any healthy habit that can be part of a normal lifestyle is going to be a winner in the long run. Anyone can do it.

It is up to you. Choose the fasting option that works best for you, and then stick to it—so the benefits are yours and stay yours.

Benefits of Intermittent Fasting

Many health benefits come from putting intermittent fasting to work in your life. In all honesty, the benefits of intermittent fasting had better be good because denying ourselves food is incredibly low on the list of fun things to do each day!

Here are the top four benefits of intermittent fasting:

1. It helps you lose weight.

2. It usually improves your brain function and mental clarity.

3. It lessens insulin resistance.

4. It usually boosts your energy levels.

These benefits blend well with all the other benefits that we have discussed earlier. The fact that our bodies can tap into these benefits by simply adjusting our eating schedule is pretty amazing.

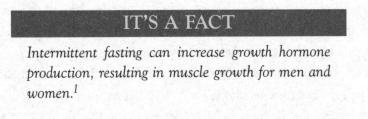

IT'S A FACT

Intermittent fasting can increase growth hormone production, resulting in muscle growth for men and women.[1]

Understanding why intermittent fasting works will help you make it a part of your lifestyle.

Along with many other medical doctors, I used to tell patients to eat three meals a day, especially breakfast as it was the most important meal of the day. Now, with the new research, we know that it's actually healthier to skip breakfast or dinner and eat only two meals a day!

The rules have changed, thanks to intermittent fasting. Some people start doing intermittent fasting one day each week and gradually move up to three to seven days each week.

Benefit 1: Weight loss

Whenever we eat, our body breaks much of the food down into glucose and stores it away as glycogen. Our bodies usually store enough glycogen from what we have eaten to hold us for around twelve hours.

That doesn't mean we won't be hungry if we don't eat; it just means our bodies are still burning sugar during those twelve hours. If we haven't eaten more food by that time, our metabolism shifts, and we begin to burn fat as fuel.

Unless we stretch the window of time in which we don't eat to longer than twelve hours, our bodies will usually be stuck in the sugar-burning mode. To tap into the fat-burning mode, we simply need to go longer between meals. And naturally, burning fat results in weight loss.

That is why some people push the 12/12 plan, the 16/8 plan, or even the 4/20 plan where twenty hours of fasting means around eight hours of fat burning. Since most people will be burning fat within sixteen hours of fasting, the 16/8 plan works well also, and many people can do this long term a few days each week.

Some studies state that the shift from sugar burning to fat burning can take place after eight to twelve hours of fasting.[2] However, I prefer to be both conservative and fat burning, so I recommend fasting for at least twelve hours.

Repeating your fasting plan of choice over and over, week after week, month after month, will help you lose weight. After all, if your body is burning fat every single day—even if it's only a little bit—over time that adds up to make a big difference.

Several years ago, the *Molecular and Cellular Endocrinology* journal compared the results of forty different intermittent fasting studies and concluded that intermittent fasting works for losing weight.[3] You would expect as much, but forty studies is pretty conclusive.

I have found some patients prefer a more traditional weight-loss plan where they reduce their daily intake of calories across the board. But for an increasing number of patients, intermittent fasting is actually easier to do on a daily basis. They don't have to count calories or buy special foods; they just manage their eating schedules.

Again, the weight-loss method you choose is entirely up to you.

On a side note, the process of burning fats rather than sugars positively impacts your heart as well. Triglyceride fats are burned up in the fat-burning process, and this directly lowers your cardiovascular disease risk![4] Intermittent fasting has been shown to also lower blood pressure.[5]

Benefit 2: Improved brain function

With the increased occurrence of cognitive diseases these days, anything that gives your brain a healthy boost needs to be seriously considered.

Like every doctor across the country, I see an increasing number of patients come into my office who battle dementia, Alzheimer's, Parkinson's, and countless other neurological challenges. The fact that intermittent fasting has been shown to reduce the risk of many neurological disorders means that everyone should pay close attention to intermittent fasting.[6]

If it helps you and your loved ones and it's admittedly easy to do, then what's the holdup?

Johns Hopkins School of Medicine professor Mark Mattson has studied decades of research on the connection between what we eat and how our brain functions. In regard to fasting and intermittent fasting, his research has found that fasting can do the following:

- help the brain ward off Alzheimer's and Parkinson's
- improve memory and mood
- protect neurons against plaque buildup[7]

In addition, David Perlmutter, MD, boldly states, "In the absence of calories, life-sustaining, protective genes responsible for cellular repair and protection are activated, inflammation is reduced, and anti-oxidative defenses are increased. This means that simply going without food for a while may have anti-aging, anti-inflammatory, and anti-tumor benefits that are available to anyone, at any time."[8]

As we have already discussed, after fasting around twelve hours the body shifts away from burning sugars and begins to burn fat. When this happens, ketones (fatty acids) are released into the blood. These ketones are an important part of losing weight.

What is more, these same ketones play a vital role in preserving your brain function, and we all want that! They even provide some protection from neurodegenerative disorders, Alzheimer's disease, and seizures.[9]

Always being a proponent of preventative medicine, I firmly believe it's better to treat an issue before it becomes a full-blown problem. Many patients who come to my office can tell their cognitive abilities are slowly becoming impaired. Seldom are neurological issues a sudden occurrence.

If you can put ketones (through intermittent fasting) to work in a preventative measure, you should do it! I have seen patients' cognitive abilities improve within a few short weeks of fasting. One study found it took only six weeks for their focus group (older adults who all suffered from mild cognitive impairment) to see memory improvement after increasing their ketone levels.[10] In fact, intermittent fasting and the ketones that work their way to your brain as a result have been found to even help new nerve cells grow in your brain.[11]

At a deeper level, ketones that are released as a result of your fasting also trigger the release of a protein called brain-derived neurotrophic factor (BDNF). What does this BDNF protein do? It "strengthens neural connections, particularly in areas involved in memory and learning"![12] In addition, BDNF has been found to help protect our brains from Alzheimer's and Parkinson's disease.[13]

Interestingly, BDNF levels can be boosted in more ways than one. Physical exercise and mental tasks will do it, as will reducing your caloric intake through fasting.[14]

Again, if something helps our brains, we really ought to do it! For our brains, working from a preventative approach is far better than waiting until the situation is dire. The fact that intermittent fasting—and fasting in general—has been found to play a significant role in helping stop, slow down, or even reverse neurodegenerative disorders like Alzheimer's, Huntington's, and Parkinson's diseases should be enough reason to take action today![15]

Benefit 3: Improved insulin resistance

The added value of lessening insulin resistance as a result of intermittent fasting may not sound all that important, but you might be surprised to learn how vital this thing called "insulin resistance" really is.

Anyone who has type 2 diabetes or who is prediabetic already knows insulin is important. However, insulin is not just important to diabetics. The very reason people have type 2 diabetes is because their bodies have become insulin resistant.

IT'S A FACT

A Hemoglobin A1C (HbA1C) test helps to determine a patient's average blood sugar control level. Your HbA1C number should be 5.6 or less, with 5.0 as the optimum. Do you know your HbA1C number?

What's happening is this: It takes higher and higher insulin levels in the blood to bind to the insulin receptors on the surface of cells so that sugar can be let inside the cells. Like a rusty lock, the insulin receptors cannot work efficiently. The key (insulin) still fits into the lock. But figuratively speaking, it doesn't turn smoothly, lots of jiggling is required, and repeated attempts with lots of other keys (more insulin) are needed before the lock will finally open.

Intermittent fasting, figuratively speaking, cleans the rust off the locks, making the insulin receptors able to receive the insulin (the key) and thereby making the whole process work much more effectively. What you want is a clean lock and a single key (lower insulin levels). It's efficient, fast, smooth, and good for your body.

Everyone alive, whether diabetic or not, requires insulin to survive. And the least amount of insulin needed to accomplish the sugar-to-inside-the-cell transfer, the better off you are in countless ways.

How then can intermittent fasting help improve insulin resistance?

First, being overweight or obese is a major cause of people developing type 2 diabetes.[16] The fact that approximately 71.6 percent of adults in the US are overweight and 39.8 percent are obese, according to the Centers for Disease Control and Prevention (CDC),[17] means that insulin resistance is important to more people than we might think and these obesity and overweight rates are going up year after year.

If hurting the body isn't enough, diabetes also hurts the pocketbook. According to the American Diabetes Association, as of 2017, the *yearly* cost of treating diabetes in the US was about $327 billion, which included medical care and lost productivity.[18] Again, that cost is per year, and it's only getting worse.

The obesity epidemic is pushing the diabetes epidemic, and it all has to do with insulin resistance. That is because every added pound makes it just a little bit more difficult for cells to operate optimally.

Men, if your waist is greater than forty inches around the navel, you are probably insulin resistant. And women, if your waist is greater than thirty-five inches around the navel, you are probably insulin resistant as well. Insulin resistance usually leads to prediabetes, and years of having prediabetes may lead to type 2 diabetes.

Insulin is important to everyone because it allows cells to take in sugar. But if your body is resistant to insulin, it becomes more difficult for sugar to enter the cells. In an effort to get sugar inside the cells, your pancreas releases more and more insulin, hoping that will help. Over time, this results in the sugar remaining in your blood because it can't get into the cell. This makes you thirsty and causes you to urinate excessively, both of which are telltale signs of diabetes. In this way, increasing insulin resistance

causes blood sugar levels to rise, and that usually means prediabetes or type 2 diabetes is on the horizon.

If insulin resistance goes unchecked or is poorly managed for
many years, the damage to the beta cells in the pancreas (the
insulin-producing cells) may be permanent, resulting in, among
other things, the need for insulin shots.

IT'S A FACT

*The longer you have type 2 diabetes, the greater your
risk of damaging the beta cells in your pancreas, which
produce the insulin your body needs. Thankfully, if
diabetes is caught early enough, you can resensitize
these insulin receptors to the point that you will not
need insulin shots.*[19]

The good news is that type 2 diabetes is fixable! I have helped
thousands of patients reverse and fix their type 2 diabetes. And
intermittent fasting can play an important role in helping to keep
your cells sensitive to the insulin your body produces.[20]

As a whole, intermittent fasting reduces the risk of type 2 diabetes because of weight loss and less insulin resistance.[21]

The weight gain/insulin resistance battle is always connected.
For that very reason, intermittent fasting is recommended for
those at risk of diabetes.[22] And if you are already type 2 diabetic,
I recommend it all the more.

Now, does weight loss lessen insulin resistance, or does less
insulin resistance bring about weight loss? The answer is yes
because it works both ways, though the greatest positive change is
a direct result of weight loss.

> ## IT'S A FACT
>
> *Insulin levels drop when you are not eating.*

We already know that rates of type 2 diabetes (among other diseases) are rising and are directly related to the obesity epidemic. Losing weight, then, will naturally help lower these disease rates.

As obvious as it might sound, if you are not eating, your body does not need to produce much insulin and your insulin levels go down. After about twelve hours of not eating, your body runs out of sugar (stored glycogen) to burn as energy and begins to burn fat and produce ketones, which help you lose weight. During this time of fasting, the decreased insulin levels may in turn cause the cells to release and therefore burn their stored sugars (glycogen) as energy.[23]

The faster the sugars are used up, the quicker your body can start burning fat as energy. That is why less insulin resistance can also boost any weight-loss efforts.

Over the years, I have helped thousands of type 2 diabetics and prediabetics reverse their symptoms and have seen hemoglobin A1C levels cut in half! With the Keto Zone diet, intermittent fasting, and some exercise (as well as hormone treatment and supplements for some), these patients have been able to get off all medications, lose weight, and restore their bodies to a healthy status.

If a person has had type 2 diabetes for longer than fifteen years, it is more difficult to reverse the insulin resistance, as the insulin-producing beta cells in the pancreas have been damaged. However, the marked improvement and many health benefits of intermittent fasting still make an amazing impact on those suffering from type 2 diabetes.

Benefit 4: Boosted energy levels

As with fasting for longer periods of time, intermittent fasting triggers something in our bodies called autophagy. This is the process of your body's cleaning out old cells, abnormal proteins, and the cellular debris built up in your system. Basically, it's house cleaning where much of the cellular trash is thrown out.

The process of autophagy does more than take out the trash and make things tidy. By cleaning out the old cells and removing abnormal proteins, the mitochondria that reside in every cell are also being cleaned.[24] In your cells, it is the mitochondria's job to produce ATP, which is your body's energy currency.

Interestingly, your heart muscle has more mitochondria than any other muscle in your body because your heart never stops pumping. Your skeletal muscles also have a lot of mitochondria, as does your liver. But stored fat tissue has very few because so little metabolism goes on there.[25]

When the mitochondria are cleaned of abnormal proteins and cellular trash, this revitalization process causes improved mitochondrial function—and that translates into more energy for your body![26]

It's exactly like a flowering bush that has been neglected. But after you trim off the dead flowers, leaves, and stems, the bush blooms all over again. New flowers appear, and the plant is healthy and happy.

If you are wondering why the mitochondria need to be cleaned up in the first place, the reason is simple: age. Blame it on the aging process, which is something that affects us all. Free radicals and disease further the damage of our mitochondria.

As we age, the mitochondria become damaged, and we accumulate cellular debris. This slows down our bodies' production of ATP, which is our energy currency.

This slowdown is painfully obvious. Compare young patients who come into my office (full of energy, a spring in their step, feeling great) with older patients (age sixty, seventy, or eighty), and the symptoms the older people complain about are *exactly* what the younger people have in abundance!

With each passing decade, energy production typically diminishes. I have seen patients at age sixty who drag into my office. After seventy, their energy is usually even lower, and after eighty, they often have hardly any energy left at all.

IT'S A FACT

Running lower and lower on energy? Your mitochondria may need cleaning, which happens with intermittent fasting.

It's the mitochondria failing to produce the energy the body needs!

When my grandson was three years old, we walked into Target together. He happened to fall behind an old man (I'd guess in his eighties) who was slowly shuffling into the store. My grandson was frustrated. He walked up to the man, hands on his hips, and said, "Why are you so slow? You are slower than a turtle." The old man laughed and said, "Son, it's because I'm so old." I apologized to the man, but he laughed again, saying, "Kids are brutally honest."

IT'S A FACT

Autophagy, as complex as it sounds, is cellular house cleaning or turning your cellular oven to self-cleaning mode. This removal of dead and old cells and proteins from your body happens when you fast. Benefits include weight loss, greater energy, less inflammation, a better immune system, delayed aging, and much more.[27]

Not long ago, I had a patient who traveled extensively overseas as a missionary. He was in his mid-seventies, was a little overweight, and was taking a lot of medications that were sapping his energy. He was so discouraged that he wanted to quit doing what he loved to do, which was to teach, preach, and minister to others.

After we met, I put him on the Keto Zone diet and recommended intermittent fasting just one day a week. He said, "That is so easy; I want to do that every day." Within a few short months of this regimen, his energy returned. He says he feels like a young man again, and his incredibly busy travel schedule is proof that it's working.

Intermittent fasting helps clear away cellular damage, which then helps repair and restore damaged mitochondria. That boosts the production of ATP, giving you increased energy, vitality, and stamina.[28]

Talking About Foods

What do you eat when doing an intermittent fast? Some say to eat whatever you usually eat when not fasting. Some allow certain snacks while fasting; others say to only drink water or noncaloric drinks. Some say to skip breakfast or dinner, while others prefer to eat their three meals anyway, just within the smaller window of time. Still others prefer a more traditional approach to fasting, going for days without any food.

You get to choose whatever fasting plan you prefer.

You also get to choose what you will eat. I recommend following the 16/8 plan as well as eating (within the eight-hour window of time) the many delicious foods listed in appendix C.

Personally, while fasting, I have found coffee with MCT oil to be a great breakfast, followed by a lunch and dinner of home-made soups that include healthy fats/oils. Snacks like celery stalks with almond butter, avocado, carrots, etc. with nuts are great to help me get through the day.

THE POWER OF INTERMITTENT FASTING IS YOURS

Intermittent fasting is a great way to get the many benefits of fasting. Yes, it's partial fasting, but it works wonders! Make it a part of your health-first lifestyle.

After all, who doesn't want these advantages?

- decreased weight
- improved brain function
- improved insulin resistance
- increased energy

Virtually every single patient who comes into my office has a sickness, disease, or symptom that is directly related to one of these four areas. Every patient not only wants these benefits but also *needs* these benefits!

Intermittent fasting can also help patients who have symptoms or a family history of Parkinson's, Alzheimer's, dementia, and age-associated memory impairment. One of my patients was a realtor, but his mild dementia forced him to quit his job. He felt like he was constantly in a brain fog, and showing up at the wrong home with prospective buyers was the end of selling homes!

He went on the Keto Zone diet, and we raised his testosterone levels to the optimum levels. But it was intermittent fasting that really brought the mental clarity he needed. His wife noted that within six weeks of intermittent fasting, his brain fog lifted and his mind became sharp again. And he went back to his real estate job.

Take advantage of intermittent fasting, and put it to work for you in your life.

You will be glad you did!

CONCLUSION

I TRUST YOU HAVE discovered that fasting is a powerful tool for health, cleansing, strength, and empowerment.

Fasting is a great way to give your body the gift of health, healing, renewed vitality, longevity, and deeper spirituality.

In this fasting program we have addressed comprehensively the wonderful benefits of cleansing the body through fasting. And I have helped you to understand the physical and other benefits of living a fasted lifestyle.

I recommend that you choose to fast periodically for detoxification purposes and that you consider intermittent fasting as more of a lifestyle to live.

If you went through the twenty-eight-day fasting program, congratulations! I commend you for your diligence and courage to establish a new health-first lifestyle plan for continued good health for you and your family.

Once you become accustomed to intermittent fasting or to fasting for two or three days, you may choose to make that a new way of living, or you may choose to increase that time a little.

APPENDIX A

RECOMMENDED NUTRITIONAL PRODUCTS

DIVINE HEALTH PRODUCTS

964 International Parkway, Suite 1630
Lake Mary, FL 32746
Phone: (407) 732-6952
Website: www.drcolbert.com
Email: info@drcolbert.com

- Green Supremefood: Ten certified USDA organic fermented vegetables and six fermented grasses (including wheatgrass, barley grass, alfalfa grass, spirulina, and chlorella), with prebiotics, probiotics, fiber, and enzymes. In apple cinnamon flavor.

- Red Supremefood: Nine certified USDA organic fruits with probiotics, prebiotics, and fiber. Delicious flavor.

- Ketozone Fiber: delicious flavored fiber with prebiotics and probiotics that support gut health.

- Beyond Biotics: My favorite probiotic and the one I place most of my patients on.

Phytonutrient powder is Green Supremefood and Red Supremefood

Enhanced Multivitamin (active forms of individual vitamins and chelated minerals)—take one in the morning

Divine Health MCT Oil Powder (french vanilla, hazelnut, chocolate, coconut cream, or plain)

SUPPLEMENTS FROM HEALTH FOOD STORE

1. Milk thistle 200 mg, two or three times per day

2. N-acetyl-cysteine (NAC) 500 mg, one capsule two times a day, or organic MaxOne, one capsule two times a day

3. Psyllium husk powder

FOOD SENSITIVITY TEST

Alcat Test (to identify food sensitivities)

Cell Science Systems

Websites: https://cellsciencesystems.com/patients/alcat-test/ and https://cellsciencesystems.com/providers/alcat-test/

The test measures non-IGE mediated reactions to foods, chemicals, and other substances. "The Alcat Test is a lab based immune stimulation test in which a patient's WBC's are challenged with various substances including foods, additives, colorings, chemicals, medicinal herbs, functional foods, molds and pharmaceutical compounds....The Alcat Test objectively classifies a patient's response to each test substance as reactive, borderline or non-reactive. Based on these classifications, a customized elimination/rotation diet may be designed to effectively eliminate the specific triggers of chronic immune system activation."[1]

APPENDIX B

DETOX RECIPES

COFFEE, TO MANY people's surprise, contains a more abundant amount of antioxidants than most any other food or beverage. Scientists have identified about one thousand antioxidants in unprocessed coffee beans and many more (hundreds) during the roasting process. Numerous studies have found that coffee is a major dietary source of antioxidants for their subjects. Coffee also helps to detox the liver, and coffee enemas have been used in many cancer clinics for decades due to coffee's ability to detox the liver and boost the antioxidant glutathione. Coffee may help prevent Alzheimer's disease (one study found that drinking three to five cups a day was associated with a 65 percent decrease in risk) and Parkinson's disease. It also helps prevent type 2 diabetes, cirrhosis of the liver, and liver cancer; reduces the risk of developing gout, and helps prevent depression.[1]

Also, according to a landmark Dutch study, moderate coffee drinkers (two to four cups a day) had a 20 percent lower risk of heart disease as compared to heavy and light coffee drinkers and nondrinkers.[2] Coffee also helps to boost short-term memory and curb your appetite.[3]

I recommend organic coffee made with alkaline water. I add one scoop of MCT oil powder to my coffee, which helps curb appetite and supports energy production and mental clarity.

If you don't like coffee, you can also drink green or black tea, either cold or hot. Add one scoop of MCT oil powder to it. (See appendix A.)

I also recommend consuming one teaspoon (level or heaping) of psyllium husk powder or keto fiber in four ounces of water or another drink, such as coffee or tea, once daily. (See appendix A.)

RECIPES FOR WEEKS 1–3

As you prepare the recipes in this section, here are some general guidelines: Use all organic ingredients, and use all fresh ingredients unless otherwise indicated. If canned foods are indicated, read labels carefully. Always use nonirradiated spices.

SMOOTHIE RECIPES

RASPBERRY SMOOTHIE

1 cup unsweetened coconut or almond milk (or alkaline water)
½–1 cup ice
¼–½ cup raspberries (fresh or frozen)
2 tablespoons cold-pressed avocado oil, macadamia nut oil, or almond oil
1–2 tablespoons avocado oil
¼–½ teaspoon organic stevia

Combine all ingredients in a blender, and blend until smooth and creamy.

BLUEBERRY SMOOTHIE

> 1 cup unsweetened coconut or almond milk (or
>   alkaline water)
> ½–1 cup ice
> ¼–½ cup blueberries (fresh or frozen)
> 2 tablespoons cold-pressed avocado oil, macada-
>   mia nut oil, or almond oil
> ¼–½ teaspoon organic stevia

Combine all ingredients in a blender, and blend until smooth and creamy.

STRAWBERRY SMOOTHIE

> 1 cup unsweetened coconut or almond milk (or
>   alkaline water)
> ½–1 cup ice
> ¼–½ cup strawberries (fresh or frozen)
> 2 tablespoons cold-pressed avocado oil, macada-
>   mia nut oil, or almond oil
> ¼–½ teaspoon organic stevia

Combine all ingredients in a blender, and blend until smooth and creamy.

BLACKBERRY SMOOTHIE

> 1 cup unsweetened coconut or almond milk (or
>   alkaline water)
> ½–1 cup ice

¼–½ cup blackberries (fresh or frozen)

2 tablespoons cold-pressed avocado oil, macadamia nut oil, or almond oil

¼–½ teaspoon organic stevia

Combine all ingredients in a blender, and blend until smooth and creamy.

LEMON SMOOTHIE

1 cup unsweetened coconut or almond milk (or alkaline water)

½–1 cup ice

½–1 whole squeezed lemon

2 tablespoons cold-pressed avocado oil, macadamia nut oil, or almond oil

¼–½ teaspoon organic stevia

Combine all ingredients in a blender, and blend until smooth and creamy.

LIME SMOOTHIE

1 cup unsweetened coconut or almond milk (or alkaline water)

½–1 cup ice

½–1 whole squeezed lime

2 tablespoons cold-pressed avocado oil, macadamia nut oil, or almond oil

¼–½ teaspoon organic stevia

Combine all ingredients in a blender, and blend until smooth and creamy.

CHERRY SMOOTHIE

> 1 cup unsweetened coconut or almond milk (or
>   alkaline water)
> ½–1 cup ice
> ½ cup cherries (fresh or frozen)
> 2 tablespoons cold-pressed avocado oil, macada-
>   mia nut oil, or almond oil
> ¼–½ teaspoon organic stevia

Combine all ingredients in a blender, and blend until smooth and creamy.

SALAD RECIPES

DR. C'S CHOPPED SALAD

> 2–4 cups romaine lettuce, chopped
> 3 green onions, chopped
> 1 celery stalk, chopped
> 1 beet, chopped
> 1 carrot, peeled and chopped
> ½ large avocado, chopped
> ½ cup chopped mushrooms
> ¼ cup chopped walnuts

Dressing

> 2–3 tablespoons extra-virgin olive oil
> 2–3 tablespoons apple cider vinegar
> Sea salt and pepper to taste

Whisk together the dressing ingredients in a small bowl. In a large bowl toss the salad ingredients with the dressing.

STRAWBERRY SPINACH SALAD

2–4 cups spinach
¼–½ cup chopped strawberries
2 green onions, chopped
1 radish, thinly sliced
½ cucumber, peeled, deseeded, and sliced
¼ cup chopped pecans

Dressing

2–3 tablespoons extra-virgin olive oil
2–3 tablespoons balsamic vinegar

Whisk together the dressing ingredients in a small bowl. In a large bowl toss the salad ingredients with the dressing.

KALE AND VEGGIE SALAD

2–4 cups (packed) torn kale leaves, stems removed
Herbamare (or sea salt) to taste
1 radish, thinly sliced into rounds
½ large avocado, chopped
½ English cucumber, deseeded and chopped
1 celery stalk, chopped
⅓ cup red onion, chopped

Dressing

2–3 tablespoons fresh lemon juice
2–3 tablespoons hemp, flax, or avocado oil

Place kale in a large bowl, and drizzle the dressing ingredients over it. Toss the dressing into the kale until all leaves are coated. Season with

Herbamare (or sea salt) and set aside, allowing the kale to marinate.

While the salad marinates, chop the radish, avocado, cucumber, celery, and onion. Mix the vegetables into the kale. Sprinkle with hemp seeds (optional) and serve.

FASTING ZONE COLE SLAW

> ¼–½ cup avocado oil mayonnaise
> 2 tablespoons apple cider vinegar
> Kosher salt and freshly ground black pepper to taste
> ½ large head green cabbage, thinly sliced
> 3 large carrots, peeled and grated
> 2 celery stalks, chopped
> ¼–½ red onion, chopped

In a large bowl whisk together avocado oil mayonnaise and apple cider vinegar. Season with kosher salt and freshly ground black pepper to taste. Add cabbage, carrots, celery, and red onion, and mix thoroughly to combine. Cover and refrigerate until ready to serve.

ARUGULA AND ASPARAGUS SALAD

> 6–8 spears asparagus
> 2–4 cups arugula
> 1 carrot, peeled and grated
> 1 radish, thinly sliced
> ¼ red onion, chopped
> ¼ cup of mushrooms, chopped

Dressing

> 3 tablespoons extra-virgin olive oil
> 2–3 tablespoons freshly squeezed lemon juice
> Sea salt and freshly ground black pepper to taste

Snap off and discard tough ends of asparagus. Slice the asparagus lengthwise into thin ribbons. Combine asparagus with other salad ingredients in a large bowl. Whisk together dressing ingredients in a small bowl. Add dressing to salad and toss well.

WATERCRESS AND AVOCADO SALAD

2 tablespoons freshly squeezed lime juice

½ shallot, minced

2 tablespoons extra-virgin olive oil

¼ teaspoon basil

Sea salt and freshly ground pepper to taste

1 bunch watercress, thick stems discarded

1 avocado, cut into thin wedges

¼ cup chopped pecans

In a large bowl combine the lime juice and the shallot. Let stand for 10 minutes. Whisk in olive oil, basil, salt, and pepper. Add the watercress, avocado, and pecans to the dressing and toss.

SOUP RECIPES

FASTING ZONE HOT AND SOUR SOUP

5 dried shiitake mushrooms

5 dried wood ear mushrooms

2 cups bone broth

1 cup water

1 tablespoon ginger, minced

1 teaspoon garlic, minced

¼ cup rice vinegar

½ cup green onions, chopped

4 tablespoons extra-virgin olive oil or avocado oil

Reconstitute the mushrooms by boiling them in water for about 10 minutes or until tender. Drain the mushrooms, slice thinly, and set aside. (You may want to save the mushroom water and use it instead of plain water in the next step for added flavor. If there is any grit at the bottom of the mushroom water, strain and discard it before combining it with the broth.)

Combine the broth, water, ginger, and garlic in a Dutch oven or stockpot. Heat to boiling over medium-high heat. Add the mushrooms and simmer 5 minutes. Add the vinegar and return to boiling. Reduce heat to a simmer. Cook for several minutes until the soup thickens slightly, stirring frequently.

To serve, ladle soup into serving bowls and top each serving with green onions and olive or avocado oil.

ARTICHOKE AND MUSHROOM SOUP

2–3 tablespoons extra-virgin olive oil
½ yellow onion, chopped
3 cloves garlic, chopped
Himalayan salt and freshly ground black pepper
   to taste
3 cups chicken stock
5–6 artichoke hearts
1–2 handfuls fresh spinach, chopped (optional)
1 cup chopped mushrooms
2 celery stalks, chopped
Pinch of thyme

In a large pot heat olive oil over medium heat. Add onion and cook until soft. Add garlic, salt, and pepper and cook 1 additional minute. Add chicken stock and bring to a simmer. Add artichoke hearts, spinach (if using), mushrooms, celery, and thyme. Allow to simmer for 10–12 minutes.

VEGGIE SOUP WITH AVOCADO

8 tablespoons avocado oil
1 cup chopped leeks (white part only)
2 cloves garlic, minced
4 cups chicken stock
3 large carrots, peeled and chopped
3 celery stalks, chopped
½ head green cabbage, chopped
½–1 cup chopped mushrooms
½ teaspoon basil
½ teaspoon thyme
Himalayan salt and freshly ground black pepper
to taste
1 avocado, thinly sliced

In a large pot heat the avocado oil over low heat. Add leeks and garlic and sauté until they start to soften. Add chicken stock and raise heat. Bring to a simmer. Add carrots, celery, cabbage, mushrooms, basil, thyme, salt, and pepper. Reduce heat to low, cover, and simmer until the vegetables are tender. Serve topped with avocado slices.

GARDEN VEGGIE DETOX SOUP

8 tablespoons avocado oil
1 cup leeks, chopped
1 tablespoon garlic, finely minced
Himalayan salt to taste
4 cups chicken stock
1 medium carrot, peeled and chopped

1 stalk celery, chopped
1 cup fresh broccoli, chopped
¼ cup fresh parsley, chopped and firmly packed
1–2 teaspoons freshly squeezed lemon juice
½ teaspoon freshly ground black pepper

Garnish (optional)

Freshly squeezed lemon juice
Fresh parsley

Heat oil in a large saucepan over low heat. Add the leeks and garlic, and sauté for 2–3 minutes. Season with salt to taste.

Add the stock, carrots, celery, broccoli, parsley, lemon juice, and pepper. Bring to a boil. Reduce heat and simmer for about an hour.

To serve, ladle the soup into serving bowls, and lightly drizzle each serving with additional lemon juice. Garnish with a sprinkle of additional fresh parsley (optional).

DETOXIFYING CABBAGE SOUP

1 pound cabbage, chopped
2 onions, chopped
2 cloves garlic, minced
2 cups beef stock
4 tablespoons extra-virgin olive oil
Himalayan salt and pepper to taste

Garnish (optional)
Fresh cilantro, chopped
Hot sauce

Combine the cabbage, onions, and garlic in a large saucepan. Add the stock and olive oil, and season with salt and pepper to taste. Bring to a boil. Reduce heat and simmer until flavors have blended, about 20 minutes.

Carefully transfer half of the soup to a blender. Secure the blender lid, and cover the lid with a clean towel and hold the lid down to avoid splattering the hot mixture. Puree until smooth, and pour into a large bowl. Repeat with the remaining half of soup. Return the pureed soup to the saucepan, and warm until thoroughly heated.

To serve, ladle the soup into serving bowls, and top each serving with cilantro and hot sauce to taste.

CREAMY CARROT AND COCONUT SOUP

2–3 large carrots, finely chopped
1 onion, finely chopped
1½ teaspoon curry powder
1 teaspoon fresh ginger, minced
1¾ cups bone broth
6 tablespoons extra-virgin olive oil or avocado oil
14-ounce can coconut milk
Himalayan salt to taste

In a Dutch oven or stockpot, combine the carrots, onion, curry powder, and ginger. Add the broth and oil, and bring to a boil. Reduce heat and simmer until the carrots are tender, about 25 minutes. Remove from heat and allow to cool for 10 minutes.

Carefully transfer half of the soup to a blender. Secure the blender lid, and cover the lid with a clean towel and hold the lid down to avoid splattering the hot mixture. Puree until smooth, and pour into a large bowl. Repeat with the remaining half of soup.

Return the pureed soup to the saucepan, and stir in the coconut milk. Season with salt, and cook until thoroughly heated.

If you choose to serve the soup hot, ladle it into serving bowls and enjoy. If you choose to serve it cold, remove it from the heat, and allow to cool to room temperature before refrigerating. Once the soup is chilled, ladle it into serving bowls and enjoy.

NOTE: Soup will thicken as it cools, so if you are serving it cold, use more vegetable broth before pureeing.

Veggie and Fruit Juices

VEGGIE COCKTAIL

> 2 carrots
> 2 celery stalks
> 1 broccoli stalk
> ½ cup spinach
> 1 lemon with peel

Juice and add 1–3 tablespoons of pulp back to the juice. Stir and enjoy!

SPINACH AND CELERY JUICE

> 1 cup spinach
> 3 celery stalks
> 2 lemons, peeled

Juice and add 1–3 tablespoons of pulp back to the juice. Stir and enjoy!

APPLE AND CARROT JUICE

> 3 carrots
> 2 celery stalks
> 1 Granny Smith apple

½ lime with peel
Handful of watercress

Juice and add 1–3 tablespoons of pulp back to the juice. Stir and enjoy!

KALE AND RASPBERRY JUICE

2 celery stalks
½ lemon with peel
½ cup raspberries
Handful of kale
Handful of cabbage

Juice and add 1–3 tablespoons of pulp back to the juice. Stir and enjoy!

BLACKBERRY BROCCOLI JUICE

½ lemon with peel
½ cup blackberries
Handful of broccoli

Juice and add 1–3 tablespoons of pulp back to the juice. Stir and enjoy!

BLUEBERRY DANDELION JUICE

2 celery stalks
½ lime with peel
½ cup blueberries
Handful of dandelion greens
Handful of watercress

Juice and add 1–3 tablespoons of pulp back to the juice. Stir and enjoy!

APPENDIX C

RECOMMENDED FOODS TO EAT WHILE FASTING

OR THE FIRST sixty days of fasting, I recommend no meats at all. That means a vegetarian diet for the most part. In his book *The Plant Paradox*, Dr. Steve Gundry provides a list of "acceptable foods" to eat at the beginning of a fast. Here are some of the foods on his list that will help your body while you are fasting.[1]

Oils:

- olive
- coconut
- macadamia
- MCT
- avocado

- perilla
- walnut
- red palm
- rice bran
- sesame

Sweeteners:

- Stevia
- Just Like Sugar
- inulin
- monk fruit
- luo han guo
- erythritol
- xylitol

Nuts and seeds:

- macadamia nuts
- walnuts
- pistachios
- pecans
- coconut
- hazelnuts
- chestnuts

- brazil nuts
- pine nuts
- flaxseeds
- psyllium

Flours:

- coconut
- almond
- hazelnut
- sesame
- chestnut
- cassava
- green banana
- sweet potato
- arrowroot

Dairy:

- coconut yogurt
- feta cheese
- goat cheese/yogurt
- sheep cheese/yogurt

Fruits:

- avocados

- blueberries

- raspberries

- blackberries

- strawberries

- lemons

- limes

Vegetables:

- broccoli

- brussels sprouts

- cauliflower

- bok choy

- cabbage

- arugula

- watercress

- collards

- kale

- kimchi

- celery

- onions

- leeks

- chives

- scallions

- chicory
- carrots
- artichokes
- beets
- radishes
- cilantro
- okra
- asparagus
- garlic
- mushrooms
- romaine lettuces
- spinach
- parsley
- basil
- mint
- seaweed

NOTES

INTRODUCTION

1. Ruth E. Patterson et al., "Intermittent Fasting and Human Metabolic Health," *Journal of the Academy of Nutrition and Dietetics* 115, no. 8 (2015): 1203–1212, https://www.ncbi.nlm.nih.gov/pmc/articles/PMC4516560/.

2. James H. Catterson et al., "Short-Term, Intermittent Fasting Induces Long-Lasting Gut Health and TOR-Independent Lifespan Extension," *Current Biology* 28, no. 11 (2018): 1714–1724.e4, https://www.ncbi.nlm.nih.gov/pmc/articles/PMC5988561/.

CHAPTER 1
THE MANY BENEFITS OF FASTING

1. "How Exactly Does Your Body Lose Water?," The Water Guy, accessed September 10, 2019, https://www.waterguys.com/blog/body-lose-water/; Emily Wax, "Water in Diet," MedlinePlus, US National Library of Medicine, July 10, 2017, https://medlineplus.gov/ency/article/002471.htm.

2. Siim Land, "Does Fasting Clear Toxins? Fasting and Detox," Siim Land, April 19, 2019, https://siimland.com/does-fasting-clear-toxins-fasting-and-detox/.

3. Rachel Hynd and NaturallySavvy.com, "Fasting Has Many Benefits for the Body," *Chicago Tribune*, February 24, 2015, https://www.chicagotribune.com/lifestyles/health/sns-green-effective-fasting-benfits-story.html; "Why Fast?," Steiner Health, accessed September 10, 2019, https://steinerhealth.org/health/fasting/.

4. Mark P. Mattson, Valter D. Longo, and Michelle Harvie, "Impact of Intermittent Fasting on Health and Disease

Processes," *Ageing Research Reviews* 39 (2017): 46–58, https://www.ncbi.nlm.nih.gov/pmc/articles/PMC5411330/.

5.   Julie Sibbing, "What's a Farm Without Fallow Fields?," interview by Alex Cohen, *NPR Day to Day*, May 6, 2008, https://www.npr.org/templates/story/story.php?storyId=90222485.

6.   Natasha Gilani, "The Effects of Synthetic Fertilizers," *SF Gate*, accessed September 10, 2019, https://homeguides.sfgate.com/effects-synthetic-fertilizers-45466.html.

7.   Don Colbert, *Toxic Relief* (Lake Mary, FL: Siloam, 2001, 2003).

8.   "Phase 1 and 2 Liver Detoxification," Digestive (Liver Detox, Nutrition, Weight Loss), CaraHealth, accessed September 23, 2019, https://www.carahealth.com/health-articles/digestive-liver-detox-nutrition-weight-loss/phase-1-2-liver-detoxification; "Allergies," Liver Doctor, accessed September 23, 2019, https://www.liverdoctor.com/allergies/.

9.   Shanshan Kong, Yanhui H. Zhang, and Weigiang Zhang, "Regulation of Intestinal Epithelial Cells Properties and Functions by Amino Acids," *BioMed Research International*, Article ID 2819154, 2018, https://www.hindawi.com/journals/bmri/2018/2819154/.

10. Enrique Cadenas and Kelvin J. A. Davies, "Mitochondrial Free Radical Generation, Oxidative Stress, and Aging," *Free Radical Biology and Medicine* 29, nos. 3–4 (August 2000): 222–230, https://www.sciencedirect.com/science/article/pii/S0891584900003178?via%3Dihub.

11. Naomi Whittel, "The 12 Important Benefits of Autophagy," Naomi Whittel, accessed September 17, 2019, https://www.naomiwhittel.com/the-12-important-benefits-of-autophagy/.

12. Mark Mattson, as told to Alexis Wnuk, "How Does Fasting Affect the Brain?," Ask an Expert, BrainFacts, July 13, 2018, https://www.brainfacts.org/thinking-sensing-and-behaving/diet-and-lifestyle/2018/how-does-fasting-affect-the-brain-071318.

13. Felice Gersh, "The Unexpected Benefits of Fasting: 3. Clearer Skin," Thrive Global, March 29, 2018, https://thriveglobal.com/stories/the-unexpected-benefits-of-fasting-3-clearer-skin/.

14. Jillian Levy, "4 Steps to Achieve Proper pH Balance," Dr. Axe, July 6, 2018, https://draxe.com/health/article/ph-balance/; Lien Ai Pham-Huy, Hua He, and Chuong Pham-Huy, "Free Radicals, Antioxidants in Disease and Health," *International Journal of Biomedical Science* 4, no. 2 (June 2008): 89–96, https://www.ncbi.nlm.nih.gov/pmc/articles/PMC3614697/.

15. Skidmore College, "Diet Helps Shed Pounds, Release Toxins and Reduce Oxidative Stress," ScienceDaily, January 11, 2017, https://www.sciencedaily.com/releases/2017/01/170111184102.htm.

16. Keld Kjeldsen, "Hypokalemia and Sudden Cardiac Death," *Experimental and Clinical Cardiology* 15, no. 4 (2010): e96–e99, https://www.ncbi.nlm.nih.gov/pmc/articles/PMC3016067/.

CHAPTER 2
ADOPTING A FASTED LIFESTYLE

1. Linlin Chen et al., "Inflammatory Responses and Inflammation-Associated Diseases in Organs," *Oncotarget* 9, no. 6 (January 23, 2018): 7204–7218, https://doi.org/10.18632/oncotarget.23208; Mark Hyman, "Autoimmune Disease: How to Stop Your Body From Attacking Itself," HuffPost, updated November 17, 2011, https://www.huffpost.com/entry/autoimmune-disease-how-to_b_283707; Donna Jackson Nakawaza, *The Autoimmune Epidemic: Bodies Gone Haywire in a World Out of Balance—and the Cutting-Edge Science That Promises Hope* (New York: Touchstone, 2008), xviii, https://books.google.com/books/about/The_Autoimmune_Epidemic.html?id=gx2apJ5MhtAC; Joseph Pizzorno, "Toxins From the Gut," *Integrative Medicine: A Clinician's Journal* 13, no. 6 (December 2014): 8–11, https://www.ncbi.nlm.nih.gov/pmc/articles/PMC4566437/; "Manifestations of Toxic Effects," Toxicology Information Brief, Extension Toxicology Network, September 1993, http://pmep.cce.cornell.edu/profiles/extoxnet/TIB/manifestations.html; Mark Hyman, "Is There Toxic Waste in Your Body?," Dr. Hyman, accessed October 1, 2019, https://drhyman.com/blog/2010/05/19/is-there-toxic-waste-in-your-body-2/; James Greenblatt, "The

Role of Heavy Metals and Environmental Toxins in Psychiatric Disorders," The Great Plains Laboratory, Inc., July 10, 2017, https://www.greatplainslaboratory.com/articles-1/2017/7/10/the-role-of-heavy-metals-and-environmental-toxins-in-psychiatric-disorders; Agency for Toxic Substances and Disease Registry, "Chemicals, Cancer, and You," Centers for Disease Control and Prevention, accessed October 1, 2019, https://www.atsdr.cdc.gov/emes/public/docs/Chemicals,%20Cancer,%20and%20You%20FS.pdf.

2. Chiara Townley, "Intermittent Fasting May Help Fight Type 2 Diabetes," Medical News Today, October 13, 2018, https://www.medicalnewstoday.com/articles/323316.php.

3. Don Colbert, *The New Bible Cure for Diabetes* (Lake Mary, FL: Siloam, 2009).

4. Bartosz Malinowski et al., "Intermittent Fasting in Cardiovascular Disorders—An Overview," *Nutrients* 11, no. 3 (March 20, 2019): 673, https://www.ncbi.nlm.nih.gov/pmc/articles/PMC6471315/.

5. Intermountain Medical Center, "Routine Periodic Fasting Is Good for Your Health, and Your Heart, Study Suggests," ScienceDaily, May 20, 2011, https://www.sciencedaily.com/releases/2011/04/110403090259.htm.

6. Geri Piazza, "Reduced-Calorie Diet Lowers Signs of Inflammatory Bowel Disease," NIH Research Matters, March 12, 2019, https://www.nih.gov/news-events/nih-research-matters/reduced-calorie-diet-lowers-signs-inflammatory-bowel-disease; Elizabeth Feuille et al., "Inflammatory Bowel Disease and Food Allergies," *Journal of Allergy and Clinical Immunology* 135, no. 2, Suppl. (February 2015): AB251, https://www.jacionline.org/article/S0091-6749(14)03541-6/fulltext.

7. Katharina Brandl and Bernd Schnabl, "Is Intestinal Inflammation Linking Dysbiosis to Gut Barrier Dysfunction During Liver Disease?," *Expert Review of Gastroenterology and Hepatology* 9, no. 8 (2015): 1069–1076, https://www.ncbi.nlm.nih.gov/pmc/articles/PMC4828034/.

8. Leila Abdelhamid and Xin M Luo, "Retinoic Acid, Leaky Gut, and Autoimmune Diseases," *Nutrients* 10, no. 8 (August 3, 2018): 1016, https://www.ncbi.nlm.nih.gov/pmc/articles/PMC6115935/; Andrea Picchianti-Diamanti et al., "Analysis of Gut Microbiota in Rheumatoid Arthritis Patients: Disease-Related Dysbiosis and Modifications Induced by Etanercept," *International Journal of Molecular Sciences* 19, no. 10 (September 27, 2018): 2938, https://www.ncbi.nlm.nih.gov/pmc/articles/PMC6213034/.

9. G. P. Lambert et al., "Effect of Aspirin Dose on Gastrointestinal Permeability," *International Journal of Sports Medicine* 33, no. 6 (June 2012): 421–425, https://www.ncbi.nlm.nih.gov/pubmed/22377941; Marcelo Campos, "Leaky Gut: What Is It, and What Does It Mean for You?," *Harvard Health Blog*, September 22, 2017, https://www.health.harvard.edu/blog/leaky-gut-what-is-it-and-what-does-it-mean-for-you 2017092212451.

10. Arndt Manzel et al., "Role of 'Western Diet' in Inflammatory Autoimmune Diseases," *Current Allergy and Asthma Reports* 14, no. 1 (2014): 404, https://www.ncbi.nlm.nih.gov/pmc/articles/PMC4034518/.

11. World Health Organization, *The Global Burden of Disease: 2004 Update* (Geneva: World Health Organization, 2008), 32, https://www.who.int/healthinfo/global_burden_disease/GBD_report_2004update_full.pdf.

12. Sharon Palmer, "Is There a Link Between Nutrition and Autoimmune Disease?," *Today's Dietitian* 13, no. 11 (November 2011): 36, https://www.todaysdietitian.com/newarchives/110211p36.shtml.

13. J. Kjeldsen Kragh, "Mediterranean Diet Intervention in Rheumatoid Arthritis," *Annals of the Rheumatic Diseases* 62, no. 3 (2003): 193–195, https://ard.bmj.com/content/annrheumdis/62/3/193.full.pdf; Chris Iliades, "How to Eat Right When You Have Lupus," Everyday Health, October 6, 2017, https://www.everydayhealth.com/lupus/eating-right-with-lupus.aspx.

14. Fiona MacDonald, "Fasting Diet Has Been Shown to Ease Multiple Sclerosis Symptoms in Early Trial," Science Alert, May 30, 2016, https://www.sciencealert.com/early-evidence-suggests-that-fasting-like-diets-could-fight-autoimmune-conditions.

15. Shigeru Nakamura et al., "Fasting Mitigates Immediate Hypersensitivity: A Pivotal Role of Endogenous D-beta-hydroxybutyrate," *Nutrition & Metabolism* 11 (August 28, 2014): 40, https://www.ncbi.nlm.nih.gov/pmc/articles/PMC4190937/.

16. Don Colbert, *The Bible Cure for Candida and Yeast Infections* (Lake Mary, FL: Siloam, 2001).

17. Rebecca Stone, "Detox With the Brown Rice Diet," SpeedyReads.com, Medium, May 17, 2016, https://medium.com/@SpeedyReads/detox-with-the-brown-rice-diet-26e85c3ecf2b.

18. Lindsay Boyers, "7-Day Brown Rice Diet," LiveStrong, August 7, 2019, https://www.livestrong.com/article/502090-7-day-brown-rice-diet/.

19. Don Colbert, *The New Bible Cure for High Blood Pressure* (Lake Mary, FL: Siloam, 2013).

20. Amy Welling, "21 Foods That Trigger Mucus Production (and 21 Foods That Reduce It)," Lung Institute, December 26, 2017, https://lunginstitute.com/blog/21-foods-trigger-mucus-production-21-foods-reduce/.

21. Don Colbert, *The Bible Cure for Colds, Flu, and Sinus Infections* (Lake Mary, FL: Siloam, 2004).

22. Corinne O'Keefe Osborn, "The Link Between Antibiotics and Yeast Infections," Healthline, March 5, 2019, https://www.healthline.com/health/yeast-infection-from-antibiotics; Jamie Eske, "What to Know About SIBO and Its Treatment," Medical News Today, February 18, 2019, https://www.medicalnewstoday.com/articles/324475.php.

CHAPTER 3
A WORLD FILLED WITH TOXINS

1. Jacqueline Krohn and Frances Taylor, *Natural Detoxification: A Practical Encyclopedia*, 2nd ed. (Vancouver, BC: Hartley & Marks, 2000), 189.

2. Krohn and Taylor, *Natural Detoxification*, 127.

3. "The Many Sources of Drinking Water Pollution," Environmental Working Group, accessed September 24, 2019, https://www.ewg.org/tapwater/sourcesofwaterpollution.php.

4. "Toxic Chemicals Released by Industries This Year, Tons," Worldometers, accessed September 9, 2019, http://www.worldometers.info/view/toxchem/.

5. K. L. Bassil et al., "Cancer Health Effects of Pesticides: Systematic Review," *Canadian Family Physician* 53, no. 10 (2007): 1704–1711, https://www.ncbi.nlm.nih.gov/pmc/articles/PMC2231435/.

6. Desert Research Institute, "Lead Pollution in Arctic Ice Shows Economic Impact of Wars and Plagues for Past 1,500 Years," ScienceDaily, July 8, 2019, https://www.sciencedaily.com/releases/2019/07/190708154038.htm; H. Abadin et al., "6. Potential for Human Exposure," in *Toxicological Profile for Lead* (Atlanta: Agency for Toxic Substances and Disease Registry, August 2007), https://www.ncbi.nlm.nih.gov/books/NBK158763/#S78.

7. Elmer M. Cranton, *Bypassing Bypass Surgery* (Charlottesville, VA: Hampton Roads, 2001, 2005), https://books.google.com/books?id=2eF8j-jlTwAC.

8. Arif Tasleem Jan et al., "Heavy Metals and Human Health: Mechanistic Insight Into Toxicity and Counter Defense System of Antioxidants," *International Journal of Molecular Sciences* 16, no. 12 (December 10, 2015): 29592–29630, https://www.ncbi.nlm.nih.gov/pmc/articles/PMC4691126/.

9. "How Common Is Breast Cancer?," American Cancer Society, January 8, 2019, https://www.cancer.org/cancer/breast-cancer/

about/how-common-is-breast-cancer.html; "Key Statistics for
Prostate Cancer," American Cancer Society, August 1, 2019,
https://www.cancer.org/cancer/prostate-cancer/about/key-
statistics.html.

10. "Criteria Air Pollutants," US Environmental Protection Agency,
accessed September 24, 2019, https://www.epa.gov/criteria-air-
pollutants.

11. Feng-You Lee et al., "Carbon Monoxide Poisoning and
Subsequent Cardiovascular Disease," *Medicine (Baltimore)* 94,
no. 10 (March 2015): e624, https://www.ncbi.nlm.nih.gov/pmc/
articles/PMC4602477/.

12. Donald Atwood and Claire Paisley-Jones, *Pesticides Industry
Sales and Usage: 2008–2012 Market Estimates* (Washington,
DC: United States Environmental Protection Agency, 2017), 10,
https://www.epa.gov/sites/production/files/2017-01/documents/
pesticides-industry-sales-usage-2016_0.pdf.

13. Michael C. R. Alavanja and Matthew R. Bonner, "Occupational
Pesticide Exposures and Cancer Risk: A Review," *Journal of
Toxicology and Environmental Health: Part B, Critical Reviews*
15, no. 4 (2012): 238–263, https://www.ncbi.nlm.nih.gov/pmc/
articles/PMC6276799/.

14. "Public Health Statement: DDT, DDE, and DDD," Agency
for Toxic Substances and Disease Registry, US Department of
Health and Human Services, September 2002, https://www.
atsdr.cdc.gov/ToxProfiles/tp35-c1-b.pdf.

15. "Dichlorodiphenyltrichloroethane (DDT) Factsheet," National
Biomonitoring Program, Centers for Disease Control and
Prevention, April 7, 2017, https://www.cdc.gov/biomonitoring/
DDT_FactSheet.html.

16. Karen Feldscher, "Pesticides Result in Lower Sperm Counts,"
Harvard Gazette, March 30, 2015, https://news.harvard.edu/
gazette/story/2015/03/pesticides-result-in-lower-sperm-counts/;
Wissem Mnif et al., "Effect of Endocrine Disruptor Pesticides: A
Review," *International Journal of Environmental Research and*

Public Health 8, no. 6 (2011): 2265–2303, https://www.ncbi.nlm. nih.gov/pmc/articles/PMC3138025/.

17. Cheryl S. Watson et al., "Xenoestrogens Are Potent Activators of Nongenomic Estrogenic Responses," *Steroids* 72, no. 2 (2007): 124–134, https://www.ncbi.nlm.nih.gov/pmc/articles/ PMC1862644/.

18. Kimberly Holland and Heather Cruickshank, "Signs and Symptoms of High Estrogen," Healthline, February 20, 2018, https://www.healthline.com/health/high-estrogen#complications.

19. Julia Phillips, "Why Fruit Has a Fake Wax Coating," *The Atlantic*, April 27, 2017, https://www.theatlantic.com/ technology/archive/2017/04/why-fruit-has-a-fake-wax-coating/524619/; "Eat the Peach, Not the Pesticide," *Consumer Reports*, March 19, 2015, https://www.consumerreports.org/cro/ health/natural-health/pesticides/index.htm.

20. S. Panseri et al., "Occurrence of Organochlorine Pesticides Residues in Animal Feed and Fatty Bovine Tissue," in *Food Industry*, edited by Innocenzo Muzzalupo (IntechOpen, January 16, 2013), https://www.intechopen.com/books/food-industry/ occurrence-of-organochlorine-pesticides-residues-in-animal-feed-and-fatty-bovine-tissue.

21. Ravindran Jayaraj, Pankajshan Megha, and Puthur Sreedev, "Organochlorine Pesticides, Their Toxic Effects on Living Organisms and Their Fate in the Environment," *Interdisciplinary Toxicology* 9, nos. 3–4 (2016): 90–100, https:// www.degruyter.com/downloadpdf/j/intox.2016.9.issue-3-4/intox-2016-0012/intox-2016-0012.pdf.

22. Kagan Owens, Jay Feldman, and John Kepner, "Wide Range of Diseases Linked to Pesticides," *Pesticides and You* 30, no. 2 (Summer 2010): 15–21, https://beyondpesticides.org/assets/ media/documents/health/pid-database.pdf.

23. Tesifón Parrón et al., "Association Between Environmental Exposure to Pesticides and Neurodegenerative Diseases," *Toxicology and Applied Pharmacology* 256, no. 3 (November

2011): 379–385, https://www.sciencedirect.com/science/article/pii/S0041008X1100175X?via%3Dihub.

24. "Groundwater Facts," National Ground Water Association, accessed September 25, 2019, https://www.ngwa.org/what-is-groundwater/About-groundwater/groundwater-facts.

25. "Technical Bulletin—Health Effects Information: Trihalomethanes," Environmental Toxicology Section, Oregon Department of Human Services, June 2004, https://www.oregon.gov/oha/PH/HealthyEnvironments/DrinkingWater/Monitoring/Documents/health/thm.pdf.

26. "Effect of Chlorination on Inactivating Selected Pathogen," Safe Water System, Centers for Disease Control and Prevention, March 21, 2012, https://www.cdc.gov/safewater/effectiveness-on-pathogens.html.

27. Stephen Gradus, "Milwaukee, 1993: The Largest Documented Waterborne Disease Outbreak in US History," Water Quality and Health Council, January 10, 2014, https://waterandhealth.org/safe-drinking-water/drinking-water/milwaukee-1993-largest-documented-waterborne-disease-outbreak-history/.

28. Sverre B. Holøs et al., "VOC Emission Rates in Newly Built and Renovated Buildings, and the Influence of Ventilation—A Review and Meta-analysis," *International Journal of Ventilation* 18, no. 3 (2019): 153–166, https://www.tandfonline.com/doi/full/10.1080/14733315.2018.1435026.

29. "Volatile Organic Compounds' Impact on Indoor Air Quality," US Environmental Protection Agency, November 6, 2017, https://www.epa.gov/indoor-air-quality-iaq/volatile-organic-compounds-impact-indoor-air-quality.

30. "Environmental Tobacco Smoke (ETS): General Information and Health Effects," Canadian Centre for Occupational Health and Safety, February 3, 2017, https://www.ccohs.ca/oshanswers/psychosocial/ets_health.html.

31. Christian Nordqvist, "What Chemicals Are in Cigarette Smoke?," Medical News Today, July 13, 2015, https://www.medicalnewstoday.com/articles/215420.php; "Harmful

Chemicals in Tobacco Products," American Cancer Society, April 5, 2017, https://www.cancer.org/cancer/cancer-causes/tobacco-and-cancer/carcinogens-found-in-tobacco-products.html.

32. "Effects of Skin Contact With Chemicals: What a Worker Should Know," National Institute for Occupational Safety and Health, US Department of Health and Human Services, August 2011, 8, https://www.cdc.gov/niosh/docs/2011-199/pdfs/2011-199.pdf.

33. Ana R. de Oliveira et al., "Chronic Organic Solvent Exposure Changes Visual Tracking in Men and Women," *Frontiers in Neuroscience* 11 (November 30, 2017): 666, https://www.ncbi.nlm.nih.gov/pmc/articles/PMC5714886/.

34. "Formaldehyde," National Cancer Institute, February 14, 2019, https://www.cancer.gov/about-cancer/causes-prevention/risk/substances/formaldehyde.

35. "Formaldehyde: Human Health Effects," Toxicology Data Network, National Library of Medicine, October 19, 2015, https://toxnet.nlm.nih.gov/cgi-bin/sis/search/a?dbs+hsdb:@term+@DOCNO+164.

36. "Phenol First Aid and PPE," Laboratory Safety Program, Cornell University, October 7, 2010, https://sp.ehs.cornell.edu/lab-research-safety/Documents/Phenol_First_Aid_and_PPE.pdf.

37. "Facts About Benzene," National Center for Environmental Health, Centers for Disease Control and Prevention, April 4, 2018, https://emergency.cdc.gov/agent/benzene/basics/facts.asp.

38. "Medical Management Guidelines for Toluene," Agency for Toxic Substances and Disease Registry, October 21, 2014, https://www.atsdr.cdc.gov/MMG/MMG.asp?id=157&tid=29.

39. "Vinyl Chloride," US Environmental Protection Agency, January 2000, https://www.epa.gov/sites/production/files/2016-09/documents/vinyl-chloride.pdf.

40. IARC Working Group on the Evaluation of Carcinogenic Risk to Humans, "2. Cancer in Humans," in *Polychlorinated Biphenyls and Polybrominated Biphenyls* (Lyon, France:

International Agency for Research on Cancer, 2016), https://www.ncbi.nlm.nih.gov/books/NBK361687/.

CHAPTER 4
A BODY FILLED WITH TOXINS

1. Ian Rowland et al., "Gut Microbiota Functions: Metabolism of Nutrients and Other Food Components," *European Journal of Nutrition* 57, no. 1 (2018): 1–24, https://www.ncbi.nlm.nih.gov/pmc/articles/PMC5847071/.

2. James Lilley, "Meet the Toxic Fungi Already Living Inside You," Medium, July 26, 2018, https://medium.com/publishous/say-hello-to-the-toxic-fungi-already-living-inside-you-c79a7bda4eb7.

3. "Acetaldehyde: Hazard Summary," US Environmental Protection Agency, January 2000, https://www.epa.gov/sites/production/files/2016-09/documents/acetaldehyde.pdf.

4. "Acetaldehyde: Frequently Asked Questions," Delaware Health and Social Services, January 2015, https://dhss.delaware.gov/dhss/dph/files/acetaldehydefaq.pdf.

5. Pham-Huy, He, and Pham-Huy, "Free Radicals, Antioxidants in Disease and Health."

6. Pham-Huy, He, and Pham-Huy, "Free Radicals, Antioxidants in Disease and Health."

7. Pham-Huy, He, and Pham-Huy, "Free Radicals, Antioxidants in Disease and Health."

CHAPTER 5
YOUR GUT HEALTH

1. Michael J. Martin, Sapna E. Thottathil, and Thomas B. Newman, "Antibiotics Overuse in Animal Agriculture: A Call to Action for Health Care Providers," *American Journal of Public Health* 105, no. 12 (December 2015), 2409–2410, https://www.ncbi.nlm.nih.gov/pmc/articles/PMC4638249/.

2. "The Central Role of the Gut," Danone Nutricia Research, accessed September 12, 2019, https://nutriciaresearch.com/gut-and-microbiology/the-central-role-of-the-gut/.

3. Robynne Chutkan, *The Microbiome Solution: A Radical New Way to Heal Your Body From the Inside Out* (New York: Avery, 2015), 3.

4. Chutkan, *The Microbiome Solution*, 94.

5. Chutkan, *The Microbiome Solution*, 11–12.

6. Warren W. Acker et al., "Prevalence of Food Allergies and Intolerances Documented in Electronic Health Records," *Journal of Allergy and Clinical Immunology* 140 (December 2017): 1587–1591, https://www.jacionline.org/article/S0091-6749%2817%2930672-3/pdf.

7. Alessio Fasano and Susie Flaherty, *Gluten Freedom: The Nation's Leading Expert Offers the Essential Guide to a Healthy, Gluten-Free Lifestyle* (Nashville: Wiley General Trade, 2014), 36.

8. Paul Rabinowitz, "Food Allergy vs. Food Sensitivity: What Is the Difference?," Allergy and Asthma Consultants, January 8, 2017, https://www.allergyatlanta.com/food-allergy-vs-food-sensitivity-difference/.

9. Rabinowitz, "Food Allergy vs. Food Sensitivity"; "5 Most Common Food Allergies People Don't Know They Have," The Wellness Way, July 29, 2019, https://thewellnessway.com/most-common-food-allergies.

10. Qinghui Mu et al., "Leaky Gut as a Danger Signal for Autoimmune Diseases," *Frontiers in Immunology* 8 (May 23, 2017): 598, https://www.ncbi.nlm.nih.gov/pmc/articles/PMC5440529/.

11. Don Colbert, *Let Food Be Your Medicine: Dietary Changes Proven to Prevent or Reverse Disease* (Franklin, TN: Worthy Books, 2016), xiii.

12. Steven R. Gundry, *The Plant Paradox: The Hidden Dangers in "Healthy" Foods That Cause Disease and Weight Gain* (New York: HarperCollins, 2017), 84.

13. Gundry, *The Plant Paradox*, 20.

14. Fasano and Flaherty, *Gluten Freedom*, 56–57.

15. University of Gothenberg, "Surface Area of the Digestive Tract Much Smaller Than Previously Thought," ScienceDaily, April 23, 2014, https://www.sciencedaily.com/releases/2014/04/140423111505.htm.

16. Jill Carnahan, "Zonulin: A Discovery That Changed the Way We View Inflammation, Autoimmune Disease and Cancer," Dr. Jill, July 14, 2013, https://www.jillcarnahan.com/2013/07/14/zonulin-leaky-gut.

17. Fasano and Flaherty, *Gluten Freedom*, 54–55.

18. "Leaky Gut: Everything You Need to Know," Rocky Mountain Analytical, March 4, 2019, http://rmalab.com/leaky-gut-everything-you-need-know.

19. Chutkan, *The Microbiome Solution*, 168.

CHAPTER 6
PORTION CONTROL

1. Elizabeth Frazão, "High Costs of Poor Eating Patterns in the United States," in *America's Eating Habits: Changes and Consequences*, Agricultural Information Bulletin no. 750 (Washington, DC: US Department of Agriculture, May 1999), 5, https://www.ers.usda.gov/webdocs/publications/42215/5856_aib750_1_.pdf?v=0.

2. Melonie Heron, "Deaths: Leading Causes for 2016," *National Vital Statistics Reports* 67, no. 6 (July 26, 2018), 8, https://www.cdc.gov/nchs/data/nvsr/nvsr67/nvsr67_06.pdf.

3. Frazão, "High Costs of Poor Eating Patterns in the United States," 5–6.

4. "How Much Sugar Do You Eat? You May Be Surprised!," New Hampshire Department of Health and Human Services, August 2014, https://www.dhhs.nh.gov/dphs/nhp/documents/sugar.pdf.

5. Brad Bloom, "Never Have a Heart Attack," CBN, accessed September 26, 2019, https://www1.cbn.com/700club/never-have-heart-attack; "Gallstones," Mayo Clinic, August 8, 2019, https://www.mayoclinic.org/diseases-conditions/gallstones/symptoms-causes/syc-20354214.

6. Richard Weindruch, "Calorie Restriction and Aging," *Scientific American*, December 1, 2006, https://www.scientificamerican.com/article/calorie-restriction-and-aging/.

7. Roy Taylor, "Calorie Restriction for Long-Term Remission of Type 2 Diabetes," *Clinical Medicine (London, England)* 19, no. 1 (2019): 37–42, https://www.ncbi.nlm.nih.gov/pmc/articles/PMC6399621/; Jean Harvey-Berino, "Calorie Restriction Is Far More Effective for Obesity Than Dietary Fat Restriction," *Annals of Behavioral Medicine* 21, no. 1 (March 1999): 35–39, https://link.springer.com/article/10.1007/BF02895031.

8. "Dietary Guidelines and MyPlate," ChooseMyPlate.gov, US Department of Agriculture, September 5, 2018, https://www.choosemyplate.gov/dietary-guidelines.

9. "When It Comes to Protein, How Much Is Too Much?," Harvard Health, May 2018, https://www.health.harvard.edu/diet-and-weight-loss/when-it-comes-to-protein-how-much-is-too-much.

CHAPTER 7
THE DETOX PLAN

1. "Nutritional Effects of Food Processing," SELF Nutrition Data, accessed September 27, 2019, https://nutritiondata.self.com/topics/processing.

2. Wendy Preisnitz, "Ask Natural Life…How Safe and Healthy Is Microwave Cooking?," *Natural Life Magazine*, accessed September 13, 2019, https://www.life.ca/naturallife/0506/microwave.htm.

3. Rollin McCraty, "The Scientific Role of the Heart in Learning and Performance," HeartMath Research Center, Institute

of HeartMath, Publication no. 02-030, 2003, 2, https://pdfs.
semanticscholar.org/7ada/8446a73a64eca9973511a8408bc21
07fc948.pdf.

4. McCraty, "The Scientific Role of the Heart in Learning and
    Performance," 2.

5. Don Colbert, *Deadly Emotions* (Nashville: Thomas Nelson,
    2003).

6. Sarah Boseley, "Poor Diet Is a Factor in One in Five Deaths,
    Global Disease Study Reveals," *The Guardian*, September 14,
    2017, https://www.theguardian.com/society/2017/sep/14/poor-
    diet-is-a-factor-in-one-in-five-deaths-global-disease-study-
    reveals.

7. Jonathan Probber, "These Tips Will Limit Cancer Risk
    When Grilling," *Chicago Tribune*, June 9, 1988, https://www.
    chicagotribune.com/news/ct-xpm-1988-06-09-8801060197-story.
    html.

8. "State of American Drinking Water," Environmental Working
    Group, accessed September 27, 2019, https://www.ewg.org/
    tapwater/state-of-american-drinking-water.php.

9. "How EPA Regulates Drinking Water Contaminants,"
    Environmental Protection Agency, accessed September 27, 2019,
    https://www.epa.gov/dwregdev/how-epa-regulates-drinking-
    water-contaminants.

10. J. Scott Boone et al., "Per- and Polyfluoroalkyl Substances in
    Source and Treated Drinking Waters of the United States."
    Science of the Total Environment 653 (February 25, 2019):
    359–369, https://www.sciencedirect.com/science/article/pii/
    S004896971834141X?via%3Dihub.

11. Don Colbert, *The Seven Pillars of Health* (Lake Mary, FL:
    Siloam, 2007).

12. Kenneth F. Ferraro, "Firm Believers? Religion, Body Weight,
    and Well-Being," *Review of Religious Research* 39, no. 3 (March
    1998): 224–244.

13. Marc Greene and Whitney Ertel, "New Research Confirms
    Green Tea Supplement Provides the Best Antioxidant

Protection," Newswise, September 11, 1997, https://www.
newswise.com/articles/new-research-confirms-green-tea-
supplement-provides-best-antioxidant-protection.

14. Sarah C. Forester and Joshua D Lambert, "The Role of
     Antioxidant Versus Pro-Oxidant Effects of Green Tea
     Polyphenols in Cancer Prevention," *Molecular Nutrition and
     Food Research* 55, no. 6 (2011): 844–854, https://www.ncbi.nlm.
     nih.gov/pmc/articles/PMC3679539/.

15. D. Pagliari et al., "Gut Microbiota-Immune System Crosstalk
     and Pancreatic Disorders," *Mediators of Inflammation*,
     Article ID 7946431, 2018, https://www.hindawi.com/journals/
     mi/2018/7946431/; "SIBO and Food Sensitivities," SIBO Doctors,
     February 2, 2017, http://www.sibodoctors.ca/blog/2016/10/28/
     sibo-and-inflammation.

16. Audrey Gaskins et al., "Effect of Daily Fiber Intake on
     Reproductive Function: The BioCycle Study," *American Journal
     of Clinical Nutrition* 90, no. 4 (2009): 1061–1069, https://www.
     ncbi.nlm.nih.gov/pmc/articles/PMC2744625/.

17. "Fiber: Why It Matters More Than You Think," Experience
     Life, April 2010, https://experiencelife.com/article/fiber-why-it-
     matters-more-than-you-think/.

18. Jill Seladi-Schulman, "What's the Length of Your Small and
     Large Intestines?," Healthline, September 18, 2019, https://www.
     healthline.com/health/digestive-health/how-long-are-your-
     intestines#large-intestines.

19. A. N. Panche, A. D. Diwan, and S. R. Chandra, "Flavonoids: An
     Overview," *Journal of Nutritional Science* 5 (2016): e47, https://
     www.ncbi.nlm.nih.gov/pmc/articles/PMC5465813/.

20. Shan Teixeira, "Bioflavonoids: Proanthocyanidins and
     Quercetin and Their Potential Roles in Treating Musculoskeletal
     Conditions," *Journal of Orthopaedic & Sports Physical Therapy*
     32, no. 7 (July 2002): 357–363, https://www.jospt.org/doi/
     pdf/10.2519/jospt.2002.32.7.357.

21. Campos, "Leaky Gut: What Is It, and What Does It Mean for
     You?"

22. Annette McDermott, "What's the Connection Between Leaky Gut Syndrome and Psoriasis?," Healthline, March 26, 2018, https://www.healthline.com/health/leaky-gut-syndrome-psoriasis#leaky-gut-syndrome.

23. María C. Cenit, Yolanda Sanz, and Pilar Codoñer-Franch, "Influence of Gut Microbiota on Neuropsychiatric Disorders," *World Journal of Gastroenterology* 23, no. 30 (August 14, 2017): 5486–5498, https://www.ncbi.nlm.nih.gov/pmc/articles/PMC5558112/.

24. "Milk Thistle," Penn State Hershey, January 1, 2017, http://pennstatehershey.adam.com/content.aspx?productId=107&pid=33&gid=000266.

25. Luca Santi et al., "Acute Liver Failure Caused by *Amanita phalloides* Poisoning," *International Journal of Hepatology*, Article ID 487480, 2012, https://www.hindawi.com/journals/ijh/2012/487480/.

26. James Meschino, "Glutathione—The Body's Master Detoxifier and Antioxidant," PDF, accessed September 28, 2019, https://pdfs.semanticscholar.org/9c25/6eb317f1d5f15cb9f59daafafd8c713568c8.pdf.

27. "Lifetime Risk of Developing or Dying From Cancer," American Cancer Society, January 4, 2018, https://www.cancer.org/cancer/cancer-basics/lifetime-probability-of-developing-or-dying-from-cancer.html.

CHAPTER 9
INTERMITTENT FASTING

1. Intermountain Medical Center, "Study Finds Routine Periodic Fasting Is Good for Your Health, and Your Heart," EurekAlert, America Association for the Advancement of Science, April 3, 2011, https://www.eurekalert.org/pub_releases/2011-04/imc-sfr033111.php.

2. Maria Cohut, "Intermittent Fasting May Have 'Profound Health Benefits,'" Medical News Today, May 1, 2018, https://www.medicalnewstoday.com/articles/321690.php?iacp.

3. Radhika V. Seimon et al., "Do Intermittent Diets Provide Physiological Benefits Over Continuous Diets for Weight Loss? A Systematic Review of Clinical Trials," *Molecular and Cellular Endocrinology* 418, no. 2 (December 15, 2015): 153–172, https://www.sciencedirect.com/science/article/pii/S0303720715300800?via%3Dihub.

4. Chris Kresser, "Intermittent Fasting: The Science Behind the Trend," Chris Kresser, March 25, 2019, https://chriskresser.com/intermittent-fasting-the-science-behind-the-trend/.

5. Kelsey Gabel et al., "Effects of 8-Hour Time Restricted Feeding on Body Weight and Metabolic Disease Risk Factors in Obese Adults: A Pilot Study," *Nutrition and Healthy Aging* 4, no. 4 (June 15, 2018): 345–353, https://content.iospress.com/articles/nutrition-and-healthy-aging/nha170036.

6. Aaron Kandola, "What Are the Benefits of Intermittent Fasting?," Medical News Today, November 7, 2018, https://www.medicalnewstoday.com/articles/323605.php.

7. Joe Sugarman, "Are There Any Proven Benefits to Fasting?," *John Hopkins Health Review* 3, no. 1 (Spring/Summer 2016), https://www.johnshopkinshealthreview.com/issues/spring-summer-2016/articles/are-there-any-proven-benefits-to-fasting.

8. David Perlmutter, "Benefits of Intermittent Fasting for Your Brain and Body," Dr. Perlmutter, November 15, 2018, https://www.drperlmutter.com/benefits-of-intermittent-fasting/.

9. Kresser, "Intermittent Fasting."

10. Robert Krikorian et al., "Dietary Ketosis Enhances Memory in Mild Cognitive Impairment," *Neurobiology of Aging* 33, no. 2 (2012): 425.e19–27, https://www.ncbi.nlm.nih.gov/pmc/articles/PMC3116949/.

11. Kresser, "Intermittent Fasting"; Mark P. Mattson et al., "Intermittent Metabolic Switching, Neuroplasticity and Brain

Health," *Nature Reviews: Neuroscience* 19, no. 2 (2018): 63–80, https://www.ncbi.nlm.nih.gov/pmc/articles/PMC5913738/.

12.   Kresser, "Intermittent Fasting."

13.   Emma Young, "Fasting May Protect Against Disease: Some Say It May Even Be Good for the Brain," *Washington Post*, December 31, 2012, https://www.washingtonpost.com/national/health-science/fasting-may-protect-against-disease-some-say-it-may-even-be-good-for-the-brain/2012/12/24/6e521ee8-3588-11e2-bb9b-288a310849ee_story.html?noredirect=on.

14.   Sugarman, "Are There Any Proven Benefits to Fasting?"

15.   Bronwen Martin, Mark P. Mattson, and Stuart Maudsley, "Caloric Restriction and Intermittent Fasting: Two Potential Diets for Successful Brain Aging," *Ageing Research Reviews* 5, no. 3 (August 2006), 332–353, https://www.ncbi.nlm.nih.gov/pmc/articles/PMC2622429/.

16.   "Risk Factors for Type 2 Diabetes," National Institute of Diabetes and Digestive and Kidney Diseases, November 2016, https://www.niddk.nih.gov/health-information/diabetes/overview/risk-factors-type-2-diabetes.

17.   "Obesity and Overweight," National Center for Health Statistics, Centers for Disease Control and Prevention, June 13, 2016, https://www.cdc.gov/nchs/fastats/obesity-overweight.htm.

18.   "The Cost of Diabetes," American Diabetes Association, accessed September 17, 2019, https://www.diabetes.org/resources/statistics/cost-diabetes.

19.   Colbert, *Let Food Be Your Medicine*, 136.

20.   Mattson, Longo, and Harvie, "Impact of Intermittent Fasting on Health and Disease Processes."

21.   Kandola, "What Are the Benefits of Intermittent Fasting?"; Mattson, Longo, and Harvie, "Impact of Intermittent Fasting on Health and Disease Processes."

22.   Elizabeth F. Sutton et al., "Early Time-Restricted Feeding Improves Insulin Sensitivity, Blood Pressure, and Oxidative Stress Even Without Weight Loss in Men With Prediabetes,"

Cell Metabolism 27, no. 6 (June 5, 2018): 1159–1160, https://www.sciencedirect.com/science/article/pii/S1550413118302535; Mattson, Longo, and Harvie, "Impact of Intermittent Fasting on Health and Disease Processes."

23.   Kandola, "What Are the Benefits of Intermittent Fasting?"

24.   Whittel, "The 12 Important Benefits of Autophagy."

25.   Miroslava Cedikova et al., "Mitochondria in White, Brown, and Beige Adipocytes," *Stem Cells International* (2016): 6067349, https://www.ncbi.nlm.nih.gov/pmc/articles/PMC4814709/.

26.   Whittel, "The 12 Important Benefits of Autophagy."

27.   Whittel, "The 12 Important Benefits of Autophagy."

28.   Daniele Lettieri-Barbato et al., "Time-Controlled Fasting Prevents Aging-Like Mitochondrial Changes Induced by Persistent Dietary Fat Overload in Skeletal Muscle," *PloS One* 13, no. 5 (May 9, 2018): e0195912, https://www.ncbi.nlm.nih.gov/pmc/articles/PMC5942780/.

APPENDIX A
RECOMMENDED NUTRITIONAL PRODUCTS

1.   "ALCAT," Perkins Chiropractic Clinic, accessed September 17, 2019, https://www.perkinschiropractic.net/wp-content/uploads/2017/04/ALCAT_INFO_UPDATED.pdf.

APPENDIX B
DETOX RECIPES

1.   Nikki Jong, "10 Healthy Reasons to Drink Coffee," One Medical, September 12, 2017, https://www.onemedical.com/blog/newsworthy/10-healthy-reasons-to-drink-coffee-2/.

2.   J. Margot de Koning Gans, "Tea and Coffee Consumption and Cardiovascular Morbidity and Mortality," *Arteriosclerosis, Thrombosis, and Vascular Biology* 30, no. 8 (2010): 1665–1671, https://doi.org/10.1161/ATVBAHA.109.201939.

3.   Jong, "10 Healthy Reasons to Drink Coffee."

APPENDIX C
RECOMMENDED FOODS TO EAT WHILE FASTING

1.   Gundry, *The Plant Paradox*, 201–203.

FREE
RESOURCE FOR YOU

Thank you for reading my book. In today's society, it's so important to know both what to eat and how to safely fast in order to cleanse your body and regain or maintain your health.

As My Way of Saying Thank You...

I am offering you a resource to help and encourage you:

- **E-book: *Stress Less*** – Printable PDF

Thanks again, and God Bless you,

Dr. Don Colbert

SILOAM